Working

As An

OperatingTheatre Nurse

The Complete Guide

ALEXANDRE CAREWELL

Table of contents

Chapter 1:
Introduction to the role
of the operating theatre nurse

Genesis of the operating theatre nurse

Let's explore the historical development of the operating theatre nursing profession. From the earliest surgical interventions to modern technological advances, this profession has undergone a significant transformation.
Historical development of the operating theatre nursing profession

The history of the operating theatre nurse goes back centuries, when the first surgical procedures were carried out in conditions quite different from those of today. Early surgical care was often performed in rudimentary environments and lacked the standards of cleanliness and safety that are now considered essential.

- **Antiquity and the Middle Ages**: During these periods, surgical procedures were often carried out by barbers, healers and religious practitioners. Post-operative care and hygiene were limited, leading to a high rate of infections and complications. Nurses did not exist as a separate profession in the operating theatre at this time.

- **19th century**: With medical advances and the emergence of asepsis and antisepsis, the role of the operating theatre nurse began to evolve. Florence Nightingale played a key role in improving hygiene practices and organising nursing care, laying the foundations for the modern nursing profession.

- **Early 20th century**: As surgery became more sophisticated, nurses began to play a more active role in the operating theatre. They were responsible for preparing patients, sterilising instruments and assisting surgeons during procedures.

11

- **Mid-20th century**: The development of modern anaesthesia and advanced surgical techniques led to a growing demand for specialist operating theatre nurses. Specific training programmes were set up to prepare nurses to work in this highly specialised field.

- **Late 20th and early 21st century**: Technological advances such as laparoscopy, surgical robotics and advanced medical imaging have transformed the way surgical procedures are carried out. Operating theatre nurses must now master the use of these technologies while ensuring patient safety.

- **Today and beyond**: The profession of operating theatre nursing continues to evolve with medical and technological advances. Nurses play an essential role in preparing operations, coordinating the surgical team, managing equipment and ensuring patient safety. They are also involved in research, training and continuing education.

In summary, the historical development of the operating theatre nursing profession reflects advances in surgery, hygiene standards and medical technology. From simple assistants in the past, operating theatre nurses have become highly specialised professionals, essential to the safety and success of modern surgical procedures.

The evolution of the role of the operating theatre nurse has been closely linked to medical discoveries that have transformed surgical practices and patient care over time. Medical advances have not only improved the safety of surgical procedures, but have also created new responsibilities and opportunities for OR nurses. Here's how medical discoveries have influenced the role of the operating theatre nurse:

Antisepsis and Asepsis: The discoveries of antisepsis and asepsis by pioneers such as Joseph Lister had a major impact on surgical care. The introduction of practices to reduce post-operative infections required the active participation of nurses to prepare and maintain a sterile environment in the operating theatre. Nurses became responsible for sterilising instruments, preparing surgical drapes and implementing strict hygiene measures.

12

Modern anaesthesia: The introduction of general and local anaesthesia has enabled more complex and prolonged procedures. Operating theatre nurses have had to adapt to carefully monitor patients under anaesthetic, manage potential side effects and work with anaesthetists to maintain patient stability throughout surgery.

Advanced medical technology: Discoveries in medical technology, such as advanced medical imaging, surgical robotics and miniaturised devices, have revolutionised the way surgical procedures are carried out. Operating room nurses have had to develop skills to handle and monitor these technologies, as well as to quickly resolve potential technical problems.

Minimally invasive surgery: The development of minimally invasive surgical techniques, such as laparoscopy, has reduced the size of the incisions required for certain procedures, resulting in faster recovery for patients. Nurses have had to learn to manage the specifics of these procedures, including assisting surgeons with specialised instruments and monitoring patients for possible complications.

Personalised medicine and genomics: The emergence of personalised medicine and genomics has led to more targeted interventions based on patients' genetic characteristics. Operating theatre nurses play a crucial role in collecting and managing relevant information to tailor care to each patient's specific needs.

In short, medical discoveries have considerably influenced the role of the operating theatre nurse, transforming him or her from a simple assistant into a highly specialised and versatile professional. Nurses must constantly adapt and acquire new skills to meet the changing demands of modern surgery and ensure the safety and well-being of patients throughout the surgical process.

The operating theatre nurse: an essential link

Operating room nurses play an essential role within the surgical team, providing specific functions and contributions that contribute directly to patient safety, efficient coordination and the overall success of the surgical procedure. Their presence and expertise are crucial at every stage of the surgical process. Here's how OR nurses contribute to the surgical team:

1. Preparation of the operating theatre: Operating theatre nurses are responsible for the thorough preparation of the operating theatre before each operation. This includes checking and sterilising instruments and equipment, preparing the sterile operating field and setting up all the necessary equipment.

2. Welcoming and preparing patients : Nurses welcome patients to the operating theatre, check their identity and medical information, and prepare them for surgery. They ensure that the patient understands the forthcoming procedure, answer any questions and allay any concerns.

3. Assistance during surgery: During surgery, operating room nurses are on the front line in assisting surgeons. They provide the necessary instruments and supplies, coordinate team members and anticipate the surgeon's potential needs. They also continuously monitor the patient's vital signs and the state of anaesthesia.

4. Instrument and equipment management : Nurses are responsible for managing sterile instruments during surgery. They hand over instruments to the surgeon according to his or her needs, monitor their use and hand them over safely to avoid the risk of contamination.

5. Documentation and record-keeping: Operating theatre nurses meticulously document all stages of surgery, including details of instruments used, actions performed and quantities of fluids administered. These records are essential to ensure traceability and continuity of care.

6. Infection prevention : Operating room nurses rigorously apply asepsis and antisepsis protocols to minimise the risk of nosocomial infections. They monitor the sterility of the environment and instruments, and ensure that all team members follow best hygiene practices.

7. Communication and coordination: Operating theatre nurses play a key role in communication within the surgical team. They facilitate the transmission of information between surgeons,

14

anaesthetists and other team members to ensure smooth collaboration.

8. Immediate post-operative care: After surgery, nurses monitor the patient closely during the recovery phase, assessing vital signs, managing pain and anticipating any side effects of the anaesthetic. They also prepare the patient for transfer to the appropriate care unit.

In short, operating room nurses bring specialist expertise and critical skills to the surgical team, helping to ensure high-quality care and a safe surgical experience for patients. Their commitment, diligence and coordination are essential to ensuring the success of every surgical procedure.

The impact of operating theatre nurses on surgical outcomes and patient recovery is significant and multifaceted. Their presence and essential role within the surgical team has a positive impact on patient safety, care coordination and the overall success of the operation. Here's how OR nurses influence surgical outcomes and patient recovery:

1. Patient safety : Operating theatre nurses play a crucial role in infection prevention, risk management and continuous monitoring of patient vital signs during surgery. Their vigilance helps to reduce intraoperative complications, minimise errors and ensure overall patient safety.

2. Adequate preparation: Operating room nurses ensure thorough preparation of the room, instruments and equipment before each surgery. Proper preparation helps reduce delays, errors and interruptions during surgery, optimising workflow and improving outcomes.

3. Team coordination: Operating room nurses act as key members of the surgical team by facilitating communication and coordination between surgeons, anaesthetists, technicians and other health professionals. Effective co-ordination allows for a better distribution of tasks, rapid decision-making and smoother management of surgery.

4. Preventing complications: Thanks to their careful monitoring and expertise, operating room nurses are able to detect signs of potential complications during surgery at an early stage. This

15

enables early intervention and measures to be taken to avoid or minimise post-operative complications.

5. Pain and comfort management: Operating theatre nurses are involved in managing the patient's pain from the very first post-operative moments. They administer appropriate analgesics and use non-pharmacological techniques to ensure patient comfort, which can contribute to a faster and less painful recovery.

6. Post-operative monitoring: After surgery, nurses continue to monitor the patient's vital signs, pain levels and reactions to the anaesthetic. Their vigilance enables any changes in the patient's condition to be detected quickly and appropriate action taken.

7. Patient education: Operating room nurses provide important information to patients and their families about post-operative care, restrictions, medications and signs of complications. Proper education promotes successful recovery by encouraging compliance and proactive health management.

In summary, operating theatre nurses play an essential role in ensuring the safety, coordination and quality of care during surgical procedures. Their contribution has a direct impact on surgical outcomes and patient recovery by minimising risks, improving the management of complications and promoting optimal recovery.

Foundations of education and training

Becoming an operating theatre nurse requires rigorous academic and continuing education to acquire the specialist skills and knowledge needed to work effectively as part of the surgical team. This training prepares nurses to take on crucial responsibilities in the operating theatre and provide high quality patient care during surgical procedures. Here is a detailed exploration of the training required to become an operating theatre nurse:

Academic training :

- **Diploma in Nursing (ASN) or Bachelor of Science in Nursing (BSN):** The first step is to complete a nursing degree, usually either an ASN which takes around two to three years to complete, or a BSN which takes around four years to complete. These programmes provide the foundations of nursing practice, including basic clinical skills and knowledge of medical sciences.

- **Licence in nursing:** After completing the nursing training programme, students must sit the national examination to obtain their licence in nursing. This licence is a fundamental requirement for practising as a nurse.

Specialised operating theatre training :
- **Operating room training programme:** Once they have graduated in nursing science, nurses interested in the operating room can follow a specialised operating room training programme. These programmes, which can vary in length and intensity, cover subjects such as asepsis, sterilisation, surgical techniques, instrument management and ethics in the operating room.

- **Operating room clinical practicum:** Operating room training typically includes supervised clinical practicums where nurses have the opportunity to apply their skills in a real operating room environment. They learn to work with the surgical team, manage instruments, participate in surgical procedures and provide post-operative care.

Continuing education :
- **Specialty Certifications:** Many operating room nurses choose to pursue special certifications to enhance their skills. For example, the Certified Operating Room Nurse (CNOR) certification is widely recognized and attests to expertise in this field.

- **Continuing education programmes:** Operating room nurses need to participate in regular continuing education programmes to keep up to date with medical advances, new surgical techniques and safety protocols. This can include online courses, conferences, workshops and seminars.

- **Advanced education:** Some nurses choose to pursue advanced education, such as a Master of Science in Nursing (MSN) with a specialization in the operating room. This training can open up opportunities for leadership, research or teaching in the field.

In summary, becoming an operating theatre nurse involves a solid academic background in nursing, followed by specialist training in the operating theatre and continuing education to maintain the skills and knowledge necessary to provide quality care during surgical procedures. The combination of these elements forms a highly skilled and competent professional within the surgical team.

Operating theatre nurses have the opportunity to pursue various specialisations and certifications to deepen their skills, strengthen their expertise and broaden their career opportunities. These specialisations and certifications allow them to stand out as experts in specific areas of the operating theatre. Here is an overview of some of the specialisations and certifications available to operating theatre nurses:

1. Certified Operating Room Nurse (CNOR) certification: The CNOR is one of the most recognised certifications for operating room nurses. It attests to skills and knowledge in surgical nursing, asepsis, patient safety and risk management. CNOR certification is awarded by the Association of periOperative Registered Nurses (AORN).

2. Certified Surgical Technologist (CST) Certification: Although this certification is generally intended for surgical technicians, some operating room nurses also choose to obtain it. The CST recognizes expertise in preparing and managing surgical instruments, assisting the surgeon and maintaining asepsis.

3. Certificate in Anaesthetic Nursing (CRNA): Although distinct from operating theatre nurses, nurse anaesthetists are often present in the operating theatre to administer and monitor anaesthesia. They are highly specialised and provide anaesthetic care before, during and after surgical procedures.

18

4. Specialisation in cardiovascular surgery: Operating room nurses may choose to specialise in cardiovascular surgery, which involves participation in complex cardiac and vascular procedures. This specialisation requires advanced skills in haemodynamics, extracorporeal circulation and the management of cardiac abnormalities.

5. Specialisation in neurosurgery: Operating theatre nurses specialising in neurosurgery work alongside neurosurgeons to assist with operations on the central and peripheral nervous systems. This specialisation requires a thorough knowledge of neurosurgical anatomy and procedures.

6. Specialisation in orthopaedic surgery: Nurses specialising in orthopaedic surgery are involved in bone, joint and soft tissue surgery. They must have a thorough understanding of orthopaedic fixation, limb manipulation and implant management.

7. Specialisation in plastic and reconstructive surgery: Operating theatre nurses specialising in plastic and reconstructive surgery assist in procedures designed to restore the form and function of body tissues. This specialisation requires special skills to work with skin grafts, implants and complex sutures.

8. Specialisation in bariatric surgery: Nurses specialising in bariatric surgery assist with weight loss procedures such as gastric bypass or gastric banding. This specialisation requires a thorough understanding of the management of obese patients and the associated complications.

These specialisations and certifications are designed to meet the specific needs of operating theatre nurses and offer opportunities for career advancement, increased recognition and the chance to contribute to specialist areas of surgery. Operating theatre nurses can choose the specialisation that best suits their interests and career goals.

Work environment and professional culture

The dynamics of teamwork in the operating theatre are essential to ensure safe, effective and successful surgery. As a complex place where several healthcare professionals work together to provide patient care, the operating theatre requires smooth coordination, clear communication and mutual trust. Here's how team dynamics work in the operating theatre:

Interprofessional collaboration: The operating theatre brings together a multidisciplinary team including surgeons, nurses, anaesthetists, surgical technicians and other specialised health professionals. Each member of the team brings unique skills and expertise, and inter-professional collaboration is crucial to overall patient care.

Defined roles and responsibilities: Each member of the team has specific, clearly defined roles and responsibilities. Surgeons lead the procedure, OR nurses assist, monitor and manage the sterile environment, anaesthesiologists are responsible for anaesthetising the patient, and surgical technicians provide technical support. A solid understanding of each other's roles promotes effective coordination.

Open and transparent communication: Communication is the key to successful team dynamics in the operating theatre. Team members need to exchange information in an open and transparent manner. This includes pre-operative communication about surgical strategy, specific patient needs and important considerations, as well as ongoing communication during surgery to share updates and resolve issues.

Collaborative decision-making: Decisions in the operating theatre are often taken in real time and may require the contribution of several team members. Collaborative decision-making enables options to be assessed quickly, problems to be solved and changing situations to be adapted to ensure the best outcome for the patient.

Managing emergencies and complications: In the event of an emergency or complication during surgery, the team must act quickly and in a coordinated manner to stabilise the patient. Each member of the team has a specific role to play in managing these situations, which requires appropriate training and ongoing preparation.

Safety culture: A safety culture is fundamental in the operating room. Team members must feel comfortable reporting potential errors, asking questions and expressing concerns without fear of reprisal. This safety culture encourages continuous learning and improved practices.

Continuous training and simulation: Continuous training and simulation sessions are essential to reinforce team dynamics. Team members can practice together in simulated scenarios to develop their communication, decision-making and emergency management skills.

In short, the dynamics of teamwork in the operating theatre are based on collaboration, communication and coordination between different healthcare professionals. Harmonious and respectful interaction between team members is crucial to ensuring patient safety, quality of care and the success of surgical procedures.

Adapting to the routines and standards of the surgical environment is an essential skill for operating theatre nurses. Working in an operating theatre requires a thorough understanding of the protocols, procedures and standards specific to this highly specialised environment. Here's how OR nurses adapt to the routines and standards of this unique environment:

1. Knowledge of protocols: Operating room nurses must be familiar with strict hygiene, asepsis and patient safety protocols. They must follow the precise steps for room preparation, instrument sterilisation, surgical drape placement and other processes to ensure a safe and sterile environment.

2. Adherence to asepsis standards: Asepsis is crucial in the operating theatre to minimise the risk of nosocomial infections. Nurses must adhere to rigorous asepsis standards, which may involve wearing sterile garments, washing hands thoroughly and using gloves and masks appropriately.

3. Cooperation in team routines: Each operating theatre has its own team routines and processes. Operating room nurses must cooperate effectively with surgeons, anesthesiologists, technicians and other team members to ensure smooth coordination and accurate execution of surgical steps.

4. Adaptation to specific procedures: Each type of surgery may have specific requirements in terms of preparation, instruments and techniques. Operating room nurses must adapt quickly to the requirements of each procedure, anticipating the surgeon's needs and providing the appropriate instruments and equipment.

5. Emergency management: Emergency situations can arise in the operating theatre, requiring rapid adaptation and a coordinated response. Nurses must be prepared to deal with situations such as haemorrhage, allergic reaction or sudden deterioration in the patient's condition.

6. Monitoring guidelines and regulations : Operating theatres must comply with strict safety, sterilisation and documentation regulations. Operating theatre nurses must follow these guidelines and ensure that all procedures are carried out in accordance with established standards.

7. Stress and pressure management: The surgical environment can be stressful and demanding. Nurses must be able to manage stress, make quick decisions and maintain concentration for long periods of time.

8. Continuing education: Adapting to the constant changes in modern surgery requires continuing education. Operating theatre nurses need to keep abreast of new techniques, technologies and best practice to ensure high quality care.

In short, adapting to the routines and standards of the surgical environment is essential for operating theatre nurses. They must master aseptic protocols, collaborate effectively with the surgical team, adapt to the specific needs of each procedure and maintain high standards of safety and quality of care.

Challenges and opportunities in the role of operating theatre nurse

Managing the stress and emotions associated with surgical situations is a crucial skill for operating theatre nurses. Working in an environment where complex medical procedures are carried out requires the ability to remain calm, focused and emotionally resilient. Here's how OR nurses manage the stress and emotions associated with their work:

1. Mental preparation: Before entering the operating theatre, nurses prepare themselves mentally by concentrating on the tasks to be performed, reminding themselves of their skills and focusing on their crucial role in the surgical team. Proper mental preparation can reduce anxiety and boost self-confidence.

2. Relaxation techniques: Relaxation techniques such as deep breathing, meditation and visualisation can help nurses reduce stress and maintain calm during stressful surgical situations.

3. Time management: Effective time management can reduce stress in the operating theatre. Nurses need to be organised and have a clear understanding of schedules and procedures to avoid unnecessary delays and emergencies.

4. Open communication: Talking openly about feelings with colleagues can help to relieve stress and gain emotional support. OR nurses often form strong bonds with team members, creating a mutually supportive environment.

5. Environmental control: Nurses can control certain aspects of their environment to reduce stress, such as soothing background music or maintaining a comfortable temperature in the operating theatre.

6. Self-care: Taking care of your own physical and emotional health is essential for managing stress. A balanced diet, regular exercise and enough sleep can help build emotional resilience.

7. Accepting imperfection: Situations in the operating theatre can be unpredictable and sometimes things don't go as planned. Nurses must learn to accept imperfection and manage challenges with flexibility and adaptability.

23

8. Professional support: Nurses may seek professional support, such as counselling or therapy, to deal effectively with work-related stress and emotions.

9. Post-operative debriefing: After a stressful or emotionally charged surgery, it can be useful for the team to hold a debriefing to discuss the emotions and challenges encountered. This can help to release emotional tension and promote a sense of closure.

Managing stress and emotions in the operating theatre is a skill that is learned with time and experience. Nurses develop personal strategies to cope with stress and maintain emotional balance while providing high quality patient care during surgery.

Operating theatre nurses have a wide range of career advancement and professional development opportunities that allow them to broaden their skills, take on increased responsibilities and explore new specialist areas. Some of the career advancement and professional development opportunities for operating room nurses include:

1. Operating room team leader: Experienced nurses can progress to team leader roles, where they supervise and coordinate activities in the operating room. They are responsible for planning schedules, managing resources and ensuring the quality of care.

2. Surgical first assistant nurse: With further training, nurses can become surgical first assistant nurses (SFANs). In this role, they work closely with surgeons to provide hands-on assistance during surgical procedures.

3. Operating theatre manager: Nurses with extensive experience can progress to operating theatre manager roles. They are responsible for the overall management of operating theatre operations, including resource planning, budgeting and process improvement.

4. Operating room trainer or educator: Some nurses choose to share their expertise by becoming operating room trainers or educators. They can train new nurses, organise continuing education workshops and contribute to the professional learning of others.

5. Specialisation in anaesthetic care: Nurses can further specialise by becoming nurse anaesthetists (RNs). They are responsible for administering anaesthesia and monitoring patients during surgical procedures.

6. Clinical research: Some nurses choose to engage in clinical research in the operating theatre, helping to develop and implement research protocols to improve surgical practice and patient outcomes.

7. Quality and safety management: Nurses can play an important role in improving the quality and safety of care in the operating room. They can participate in continuous improvement initiatives, analyse data and implement best practices.

8. Teaching and training: Some nurses choose to become teachers of nursing or surgical care in training schools. They share their expertise with the next generation of operating theatre nurses.

9. Consulting or advising: Experienced nurses may work as independent consultants or advisers for pharmaceutical companies, medical device companies or healthcare organisations, sharing their expertise in the operating theatre.

10. Developing a specialist career: Nurses may choose to specialise in specific areas of surgery, such as cardiovascular surgery, neurosurgery, orthopaedic surgery, plastic surgery, etc. This expertise can open up unique and rewarding opportunities. This expertise can open up unique and rewarding opportunities.

In short, OR nurses have many opportunities for career advancement and professional development that allow them to progress, specialise and have a significant impact on surgical care and patient safety. These opportunities reflect the diversity of skills and interests within the OR nursing profession.

Professional ethics and values

Fundamental ethical principles play an essential role in the surgical context, where operating theatre nurses are faced with complex decisions that have a direct impact on patients' lives and health. Respecting these ethical principles is crucial to ensuring high quality care, patient safety and maintaining professional integrity. Here are some of the fundamental ethical principles that guide operating theatre nurses:

1. Patient autonomy : Respect for patient autonomy is a key ethical principle. Nurses must inform patients about their condition, treatment options and associated risks, so that they can make informed decisions and consent to surgical procedures. This requires open and honest communication.

2. Caring: Operating room nurses have an ethical responsibility to maintain patient well-being and comfort at all times. This includes taking steps to alleviate pain, reduce anxiety and respect the patient's dignity during surgical procedures.

3. Non-maleficence: The principle of non-maleficence requires operating room nurses to take steps to avoid causing unnecessary or avoidable harm to patients. This includes implementing safety practices, preventing infections and proactively managing potential complications.

4. Patient benefit : Nurses must act in the best interests of the patient, ensuring that decisions made and actions taken have the patient's welfare as their primary objective. This may involve questioning decisions that are not in the patient's best interests.

5. Justice: Justice requires that operating room nurses treat all patients equally, without discrimination or prejudice. This includes fair access to surgical care and fair distribution of resources.

6. Confidentiality: Nurses must respect the confidentiality of patients' medical information, including details of their health condition and medical history. This helps to build trust between the patient and the care team.

7. Professional integrity: Operating room nurses must maintain high standards of professional integrity. This includes honesty, transparency, compliance with rules and regulations, and the recognition and management of potential conflicts of interest.

8. Respect for privacy: In addition to confidentiality, nurses must respect patients' privacy by providing respectful care and preserving their dignity during surgical procedures.

9. Accountability: Operating room nurses are accountable for their actions and decisions. They must be prepared to be accountable for their choices and take responsibility for the consequences of their actions.

10. Continuing education and professional development: Operating theatre nurses have an ethical obligation to continue their continuing education and professional development in order to keep their skills up to date and ensure high quality care.

In short, fundamental ethical principles guide operating room nurses in making complex and delicate decisions. By respecting these principles, nurses contribute to improving surgical care, ensuring patient safety and maintaining public confidence in the nursing profession.

Respect for confidentiality, informed consent and patients' rights is an essential aspect of operating theatre nursing practice. These ethical and legal principles aim to protect patients' dignity, privacy and choice throughout the surgical process. Here's how OR nurses strive to respect these crucial elements:

1. Maintaining confidentiality: Operating room nurses are required to maintain the confidentiality of patients' medical information. This means that they must not disclose details of a patient's medical condition, medical history or any other personal information to unauthorised third parties. Confidentiality is essential to establish trust between the patient and the care team, as well as to comply with legal and ethical standards.

2. Informed consent: Operating room nurses play a crucial role in the informed consent process. They must ensure that the patient fully understands the details of the surgical procedure, including the risks, benefits and possible alternatives. Nurses can help clarify information, answer the patient's questions and facilitate communication between the patient and the surgeon. Informed consent ensures that the patient makes an informed and voluntary decision about their treatment.

3. Respect for patients' rights : Operating room nurses must respect patients' fundamental rights, such as the right to dignity, privacy, autonomy and respect. This means treating each patient with compassion, respecting their cultural and religious preferences, and taking into account their individual needs during the surgical procedure.

4. Empathetic communication: Operating theatre nurses must communicate empathetically with patients and their families. They can be present to reassure and emotionally support patients before surgery, addressing their concerns and providing a safe space to express their emotions.

5. Privacy: In the operating theatre, nurses should take steps to protect patient privacy during preparations and procedures. This may include draping the patient appropriately and minimising irrelevant personal conversations.

6. Incorporation of advance directives : Nurses should ensure that the patient's advance directives, such as end-of-life wishes or medical preferences, are respected during the surgical procedure. This may involve working with the surgical team to ensure that the patient's choices are honoured.

7. Protection of medical information: Nurses must ensure that patients' medical records and sensitive information are stored securely and are only accessible to authorised persons. This helps to prevent breaches of confidentiality and invasions of privacy.

In short, respect for confidentiality, informed consent and patient rights are at the heart of the ethical practice of operating theatre nurses. These principles ensure that patients are treated with dignity, respect and integrity throughout their surgical journey, and reinforce trust between patients, families and the care team.

Expectations for future operating theatre nurses in terms of knowledge and skills are high due to the complex and specialised nature of this field. Operating theatre nurses play a crucial role in delivering safe, high quality surgical care to patients. The following are the key knowledge and skills expectations for future operating theatre nurses:

1. In-depth knowledge of anatomy and physiology: Future operating room nurses must have a solid understanding of the anatomy and physiology of the human body. This enables them to understand anatomical structures, physiological functions and the implications for surgical procedures.

2. Mastery of sterilisation and asepsis techniques: Operating theatre nurses must be experts in sterilisation, disinfection and asepsis techniques to maintain a sterile environment and prevent nosocomial infections.

3. Technical and instrumentation skills: Nurses must be competent in the handling and maintenance of surgical instruments, equipment and technologies used in the operating theatre.

4. Knowledge of surgical procedures: They must have a thorough understanding of the different surgical procedures, the steps involved, the instruments needed and the specific roles of each member of the surgical team.

5. Communication and coordination skills: Future operating theatre nurses must be excellent communicators and coordinators. They must be able to work effectively with team members, relay information clearly and accurately and maintain open communication during procedures.

6. Emergency management: Operating room nurses must be prepared to manage emergencies and complications that may arise during surgery.

7. Ethics and respect for patients' rights : Future nurses must be aware of the ethical principles relating to confidentiality, informed consent, patient dignity and respect for patients' rights.

8. Adaptability and resilience: Working in the operating theatre can be unpredictable and demanding. Nurses must be able to adapt to change, manage stress and remain calm under pressure.

9. Continuing education and updating skills: Expectations for operating theatre nurses are changing as medical and technological advances are made. Future nurses must be committed to continuing education and be prepared to acquire new skills to keep up to date.

In short, future operating room nurses must possess a solid base of medical knowledge, advanced technical skills and the human qualities essential to providing high-quality care in a surgical environment. The combination of these knowledge and skills will prepare them to succeed in this demanding and rewarding area of nursing practice.

Chapter 2:
Preparation before surgery

Planning and coordination of the surgical day

Scheduling operations and managing the surgical calendar are key responsibilities for operating theatre nurses. These tasks require careful planning, effective coordination and transparent communication to ensure that surgical procedures run smoothly and resources are used to best effect. Here's how nurses manage these critical aspects:

Establishing the order of operations :
- **Coordination with the medical team:** Operating room nurses work with surgeons, anaesthetists, residents and other members of the medical team to establish the order of operations. This coordination ensures that each operation is planned according to the team's availability and the resources required.

- **Prioritising cases: Depending on** the complexity of the procedure, the patient's condition and other factors, nurses assess the priority of surgical cases. Emergency cases and higher-risk patients may be scheduled first.

- **Optimisation of resources:** The order of operations is also established taking into account the estimated duration of each operation, the availability of operating theatres, the necessary staff and specialised equipment.

- **Planning staff changes:** Nurses need to take into account staff changeover and break periods when establishing the order of operations. This ensures that the team remains energetic and focused throughout the day.

Surgical schedule management :
- **Long-term planning:** Operating room nurses participate in long-term planning of the surgical calendar, taking into account requests for elective surgery, available resources and patient needs.

- **Booking operating theatres:** They coordinate with the operating theatre managers to book the operating theatres according to the order of operations and the time slots available.

- **Communication with patients:** Operating theatre nurses can play a role in communicating with patients to arrange dates for surgery, explain preoperative preparations and answer questions.

- **Real-time adaptation:** During the day, nurses monitor the progress of operations, react to emergencies and unforeseen schedule changes, and ensure agile management of the surgical calendar.

- **Reducing delays:** Effective management of the surgical calendar helps to minimise delays, which is crucial to optimising the use of time in the operating theatre and reducing the impact on patients and staff.

- **Precise documentation:** Operating theatre nurses keep detailed records of procedures carried out, start and finish times, teams involved and any significant events.

Scheduling operations and managing the surgical calendar requires strategic planning, transparent communication and the ability to adapt to changes in real time. Operating room nurses play a central role in these critical aspects to ensure efficient workflow, optimal use of resources and delivery of high quality patient care.

Communication with the medical team is of crucial importance for operating theatre nurses, as it ensures a smooth transition between the different phases of a surgical operation. Clear, open and effective communication helps to ensure patient safety, the coordination of tasks and the smooth running of the procedure. Here's how OR nurses manage communication with the medical team:

1. Pre-operative briefing: Before the start of each operation, the medical team, including surgeons, anaesthetists, nurses and technicians, meet for a pre-operative briefing. During this meeting, the roles and responsibilities of each team member are clarified, details of the procedure are discussed, and any concerns or questions are addressed. This ensures that all team members have a common understanding of what needs to be done.

2. Transmission of essential information: Operating theatre nurses are responsible for the transmission of essential information between members of the medical team. This may include details of the patient's condition, medical history, allergies, results of pre-operative tests and other relevant information.

3. Status reports: During surgery, nurses can provide regular status reports to the medical team, indicating the steps reached, the next steps planned and important events that have occurred during the procedure. These updates help maintain a real-time understanding of the situation.

4. Non-verbal communication: In addition to verbal communication, operating theatre nurses also use codified signals and gestures to facilitate communication in an environment where ambient noise can be high and sterility must be maintained.

5. Emergency management: In the event of complications or emergencies during the procedure, operating theatre nurses work closely with members of the medical team to make rapid and effective decisions to stabilise the patient.

6. Communication with patients : Nurses can also play a role in communicating with patients, answering their questions, reassuring them and explaining the steps of the procedure in an understandable way.

7. Post-operative debriefing: After surgery, the medical team participates in a post-operative debriefing to discuss how the procedure went, share observations and lessons learned, and identify opportunities for improvement.

Transparent and collaborative communication between nurses and members of the medical team promotes a safe working environment, reduces errors and risks, and contributes to high quality surgical care. It's an essential aspect of operating theatre practice that strengthens the coordination, mutual trust and efficiency of the medical team.

Preparing facilities and the environment

Preparing the operating theatre is a crucial step in the surgical process, and operating theatre nurses play a vital role in this task. Careful and methodical preparation of the operating theatre ensures a sterile, safe and well-organised environment for surgical procedures. Here's how operating theatre nurses prepare the operating theatre:

1. Disinfection and asepsis :
- Operating theatre nurses follow strict disinfection and asepsis protocols to prevent nosocomial infections and maintain a sterile environment. They thoroughly clean and disinfect all surfaces in the operating theatre, including operating tables, equipment, instruments and trolleys.

- Surfaces and equipment that must remain sterile are covered with sterile sheets or surgical drapes, which are carefully laid out to avoid contamination.

2. Preparation of instruments and materials :
- Operating theatre nurses check and prepare all the instruments, surgical tools and medical equipment needed for the procedure. They ensure that everything is sterile, works properly and is accessible to the surgical team.

- Sterile instruments are placed on pre-prepared instrument tables in the order required for the procedure. Each instrument is checked against the preoperative list to avoid errors.

3. Preparation of solutions and products :
- Operating theatre nurses prepare the antiseptic solutions, medicines and products required for the procedure. They ensure that medicines are correctly labelled and prepared in accordance with safety protocols.

4. Checking equipment :
- Before the procedure begins, the operating theatre nurses check that all the equipment, such as monitors, operating lights, aspirators, anaesthesia machines, etc., are working properly and ready to be used.

5. Preparing the patient :
- Operating room nurses prepare the patient by placing sterile drapes over the operating area and positioning the patient in accordance with the requirements of the surgical procedure. They also ensure that the patient is correctly identified and that all the necessary medical information is available.

6. Team check :
- Before the patient arrives, the surgical team, including nurses, surgeons and anaesthetists, carry out a final check of everything, including sterility, the layout of instruments and equipment, and the details of the procedure.

Meticulous preparation of the operating theatre ensures a safe, sterile and well-organised environment for surgical procedures. Operating theatre nurses ensure that all the necessary elements are in place, that safety protocols are followed and that the team is ready to provide high quality surgical care to patients.

Checking the availability and functionality of medical equipment is an essential step in preparing the operating theatre and ensuring patient safety during surgery. Operating theatre nurses play a central role in this task, which aims to ensure that all the necessary equipment is operational and ready for use. Here's how nurses carry out this critical check:

1. Preoperative inspection :
- Before the patient arrives in the operating theatre, the nurses carry out a complete inspection of the theatre and the equipment. They check that all apparatus, monitors, surgical instruments, operating lights, anaesthetic machines and other equipment are present and correctly installed.

2. Checking calibrations and settings :
- Nurses ensure that the necessary equipment is calibrated and set to the required specifications. This may include checking the accuracy of monitors, pressure systems, temperatures, flow rates and other vital parameters.

3. Function testing :
  - Every piece of equipment is tested to ensure that it is working properly. Nurses check that all buttons, controls and displays are operational and respond to commands. Safety and emergency stop devices are also tested.

4. Preparing consumables :
  - The nurses ensure that all the necessary consumables, such as infusion supplies, syringes, medicines, antiseptic solutions, sterile sheets, etc., are available and ready to use.

5. Communication with the team :
  - If any problems or concerns about the equipment are identified, the nurses immediately inform the other members of the surgical team, including the surgeons and anaesthetists. This allows any potential problems to be resolved quickly before the procedure begins.

6. Documentation :
  - All stages of equipment verification are carefully documented. This includes test results, corrections made in the event of a problem, and any other relevant information.

7. Further training :
  - Operating theatre nurses take part in ongoing training to keep abreast of the latest technological advances, new procedures for using equipment and best practice in medical device safety.

Checking the availability and functionality of medical equipment is a fundamental step in ensuring patient safety and the smooth running of surgical procedures. Operating theatre nurses play an essential role in this task by ensuring that all the necessary equipment is in perfect working order and ready to be used to provide high-quality care.

Preparing the patient for surgery

The pre-operative assessment is a crucial step in preparing a patient for surgery. Operating theatre nurses play an essential role in this assessment by gathering relevant medical information to ensure the patient's safety during the procedure. Here's how nurses conduct a comprehensive pre-operative assessment:

1. Taking a medical history :
   - Operating theatre nurses interview the patient to gather detailed information about their medical history. This includes a history of illnesses, pre-existing medical conditions, previous surgical procedures, hospitalisations, allergies, past medical treatments and previous medical test results.

2. Allergy check :
   - The nurses ensure that all the patient's allergies are identified, whether they be drug allergies, food allergies or other allergies. This information is vital to avoid any allergic reactions during the procedure and to ensure that the medicines and products used are safe for the patient.
   -

3. Review of medicines :
   - Nurses carefully examine the list of medicines the patient takes regularly. This includes prescription drugs, over-the-counter medicines, supplements and herbal remedies. This assessment is important to avoid drug interactions and to adjust medication as needed during and after surgery.
   -

4. Assessment of risk factors :
   - Operating theatre nurses identify potential risk factors associated with the patient, such as hypertension, diabetes, heart problems, smoking, etc. These factors are taken into account to plan appropriate monitoring and treatment measures during and after the procedure. These factors are taken into account to plan appropriate monitoring and treatment measures during and after the procedure.
   -

5. Assessment of vital functions :
   - Nurses monitor the patient's vital signs, including heart rate, blood pressure, temperature and oxygen saturation. This assessment is used to detect any significant changes in the patient's condition.
   -

6. Preparing the patient :
   - Depending on the results of the pre-operative assessment, nurses may take steps to optimise the patient's condition

before surgery. This may include managing medication, correcting electrolyte imbalances, stabilising blood pressure, etc.

7. Communication with the medical team :
   - The results of the pre-operative assessment are communicated to the surgical team, including the surgeons, anaesthetists and other health professionals involved. This information helps to make informed decisions about the conduct of the procedure.

Pre-operative assessment enables operating theatre nurses to gather essential information to ensure patient safety during the surgical procedure. A thorough and accurate assessment contributes to personalised patient care, preventing complications and optimising surgical results.

The physical preparation of the patient prior to surgery is a vital step in ensuring the success of the procedure and minimising potential risks. Operating theatre nurses play an essential role in this preparation by ensuring that the patient follows the appropriate protocols to guarantee a sterile and safe environment. Here's how nurses handle the physical preparation of the patient:

1. Preoperative fasting :
   - Operating theatre nurses provide specific instructions to the patient regarding pre-operative fasting, including the period of time during which the patient must refrain from eating and drinking. Fasting is essential to reduce the risk of regurgitation and aspiration during anaesthesia.

2. Skin preparation and body hygiene :
   - The nurses explain to the patient how to prepare the skin properly, generally using antiseptic products. Clean, disinfected skin reduces the risk of post-operative infection. The patient may be asked to take a shower or to clean the operating area with a specific disinfectant product.

3. Dressing for surgery :
   - Before entering the operating theatre, the patient is dressed in sterile surgical clothing. Nurses assist the

patient in this process to ensure that all exposed areas are covered with sterile drapes. This helps to maintain a sterile environment during the procedure.

4. Removal of jewellery and personal items :
   - Nurses advise patients to remove all jewellery, piercings and personal items before surgery. This reduces the risk of contamination and avoids interference with medical equipment.

5. Answers to the patient's questions :
   - The nurses answer the patient's questions and concerns about physical preparation and the forthcoming procedure. They ensure that the patient understands the instructions and is mentally ready for the procedure.

6. Communication with the anaesthetist and surgical team :
   - The nurses communicate the details of the patient's physical preparation to the anaesthetist and the surgical team. This information is taken into account when planning the anaesthetic and the procedure.

Proper physical preparation of the patient is essential to ensure a sterile, safe and well-organised environment in the operating theatre. Operating theatre nurses guide the patient through these critical steps, ensuring that protocols are followed, that the patient is comfortable and that all necessary steps are taken for a safe and successful surgery.

Anaesthesia and sedation procedures

Preparing anaesthetic equipment and assisting the anaesthetist are crucial aspects of preparing an operating theatre for surgery. Operating theatre nurses play an essential role in these tasks, working closely with the anaesthetist to ensure patient safety and comfort during the procedure. Here's how nurses deal with preparing anaesthetic equipment and assisting the anaesthetist:

1. Preparation of anaesthetic equipment :
   - Operating theatre nurses work with the anaesthetist to prepare the anaesthetic equipment needed for the procedure. This includes anaesthetic drugs, endotracheal

tubes, intravenous catheters, vital sign monitors, face masks, tubing and other related equipment.

2. Checking and calibrating equipment :
   - Nurses ensure that all anaesthetic equipment is checked, calibrated and ready for use. They check the accuracy of monitors, ventilation devices, anaesthesia machines and infusion pumps.
   •

3. Assistance to the anaesthetist :
   - During the administration of anaesthesia, nurses assist the anaesthetist by carefully monitoring the patient, helping to position the patient appropriately and providing the necessary instruments and equipment.

4. Preparation of the injection and infusion site :
   - Nurses prepare the injection site for anaesthetic drugs and insert intravenous catheters to ensure access to drugs and intravenous fluids during the procedure.

5. Psychological support for the patient :
   - Nurses provide psychological support to patients by explaining the anaesthetic process, answering questions and helping them to relax before the procedure.

6. Communication with the surgical team :
   - The nurses communicate regularly with the surgical team, including the surgeons, to ensure that the patient is ready for the operation and that all aspects relating to anaesthesia are taken into account.

7. Precise documentation :
   - Operating theatre nurses accurately document every detail of the preparation of anaesthetic equipment, the drugs administered and the monitoring of the patient during the procedure.

Assisting the anaesthetist and preparing the anaesthetic equipment are essential to ensure patient safety during the surgical procedure. Operating theatre nurses play a key role in ensuring that all aspects of anaesthesia are carefully planned, executed and monitored to provide safe, high quality care.

Monitoring vital signs during induction of anaesthesia is a critical step in ensuring patient safety and monitoring response to anaesthetic agents. Operating theatre nurses play an essential role in this continuous monitoring to detect any potentially dangerous changes and act quickly if necessary. Here's how nurses monitor vital signs during induction of anaesthesia:

1. Continuous monitoring :
   - Nurses constantly monitor the patient's vital signs during the induction of anaesthesia. This includes heart rate, blood pressure, respiratory rate, oxygen saturation, body temperature and other important parameters.

2. Use of monitors :
   - Nurses use advanced medical monitors to monitor a patient's vital signs in real time. These monitors provide accurate, continuous data to help detect any abnormal changes quickly.

3. Reaction to anaesthesia :
   - Nurses monitor the patient's response to the administration of anaesthetic, including variations in heart rate, blood pressure and oxygen saturation.

4. Response to interventions :
   - If the patient's vital signs show significant or unexpected changes, nurses react immediately by taking measures to stabilise the patient. This may include adjusting ventilation, administering medication, increasing oxygen supply or other necessary interventions.

5. Communication with the anaesthetist :
   - Operating theatre nurses are in constant communication with the anaesthetist to share information on vital sign monitoring and to discuss any concerns or needs for intervention.

6. Precise documentation :
   - All data relating to the monitoring of vital signs is carefully documented. This includes baseline values, variations observed, interventions undertaken and patient response.

7. Post-induction monitoring :
 • Monitoring of vital signs continues after induction of anaesthesia to ensure that the patient remains stable throughout the surgical procedure.

Continuous monitoring of vital signs during induction of anaesthesia is essential to ensure patient safety and well-being throughout the surgical procedure. Operating theatre nurses play a critical role in carefully monitoring vital signs, identifying abnormal changes and taking appropriate action to maintain patient stability and ensure high quality care.

Verification of documents and informed consent

Checking medical records, informed consents and surgical protocols is an essential step in preparing for surgery. Operating theatre nurses play a key role in this check to ensure that all the necessary information is correct, that the patient is well informed and that safety protocols are followed. Here's how they do it:

1. Checking medical records :
 • Operating theatre nurses carefully review the patient's medical records to ensure that all relevant medical information is correct and up to date. This includes medical history, test results, allergies, medications taken, consultation notes and any other relevant information.

2. Verification of informed consent :
 • Nurses confirm that the patient has signed an informed consent for the surgical procedure. They ensure that the consent is complete, dated and signed in accordance with legal and ethical requirements.

3. Compliance with surgical protocols :
 • Operating room nurses ensure that surgical protocols specific to the procedure are followed. This may include specific patient preparation, required pre-operative steps, sterilisation and asepsis protocols, and other specific guidelines.

4. Communication with the surgical team :
  - If discrepancies or inconsistencies are identified in medical records, informed consents or surgical protocols, the nurses immediately inform the surgical team, including the surgeons and anaesthetists. This allows any problems to be resolved before the procedure begins.

5. Final team check :
  - Before the operation begins, the surgical team, including nurses, surgeons and anaesthetists, carry out a final check of everything, including medical records, informed consents and surgical protocols.

6. Precise documentation :
  - All stages of the audit are carefully documented. This includes the checks carried out, the results, the actions taken and communications with the surgical team.

Rigorous verification of medical records, informed consents and surgical protocols is essential to ensure patient safety, regulatory compliance and the smooth running of the surgical procedure. Operating theatre nurses play a crucial role in ensuring that all information is correct, that the patient is well informed and that safety protocols are strictly followed.

Preventing medical errors and communication problems is of crucial importance in the operating theatre to ensure patient safety and the quality of surgical care. Operating room nurses play an essential role in implementing protocols and practices to minimise errors and improve communication within the surgical team. Here's how nurses help prevent medical errors and improve communication:

1. Cross-checking information :
  - Operating theatre nurses carry out rigorous cross-checks to ensure that patient information, planned procedures and drugs administered are correct. They confirm critical details with the surgical team to avoid errors.

2. Use of checklists :
  - Nurses follow specific checklists for each stage of the surgical procedure, from preparation to closure. These lists

help to ensure that all the necessary tasks are completed and that nothing is omitted.

3. Open and transparent communication :
   - Nurses encourage open and transparent communication within the surgical team. They share relevant information, ask questions and express concerns to avoid misunderstandings.

4. Use of effective communication tools :
   - Nurses use communication tools such as whiteboards, e-mail systems and X-rays to keep in touch with members of the surgical team and exchange important information in real time.

5. Clarification of medical orders :
   - If something seems ambiguous or inaccurate in the medical orders, the nurses ask the anaesthetist or surgeon for clarification to avoid any confusion.

6. Using the SBAR method :
   - Nurses frequently use the SBAR (Situation, Background, Assessment, Recommendation) method to structure important communications with the surgical team, providing clear and concise information.

7. Communication training :
   - Nurses take part in interprofessional communication training to improve their communication skills and learn to work effectively as part of a team.

8. Analysis of errors and incidents :
   - Nurses take part in analyses of errors and incidents that occur in the operating theatre. This enables the root causes to be identified and preventive measures to be put in place to avoid repetition.

Preventing medical errors and communication problems relies on a culture of safety, open communication and constant vigilance. Operating room nurses play a key role by being advocates for patient safety, monitoring processes, reporting problems and contributing to the continuous improvement of surgical practices.

Managing emergencies and unforeseen events

Preparing for emergency scenarios is an essential part of the operating theatre nurse's role. Although surgical procedures are meticulously planned, emergencies can occur at any time. Nurses must be prepared to react quickly and effectively to ensure patient safety and the best possible outcome. Here's how nurses prepare for emergency scenarios such as cardiac arrest and excessive bleeding:

1. Advanced life support training :
   - Operating theatre nurses are trained in advanced resuscitation, including cardiopulmonary resuscitation (CPR) techniques, the use of defibrillators and other skills needed to manage cardiac arrest.

2. Established emergency protocols :
   - Nurses are familiar with the emergency protocols established for different scenarios, such as cardiac arrest, excessive bleeding, anaphylaxis, etc. They know the steps to follow and the specific roles of each team member. They know the steps to follow and the specific roles of each team member.

3. Preparing emergency equipment :
   - Nurses ensure that emergency equipment, such as resuscitation trolleys, intubation kits, bleeding tamponade devices and emergency medicines, are ready for use and easily accessible when needed.

4. Fast communication :
   - In the event of an emergency scenario, nurses communicate rapidly with the surgical team, including surgeons, anaesthetists and other health professionals, to coordinate actions and interventions.

5. Stress management :
   - Nurses are trained to manage stress in emergency situations. They maintain their composure, make informed decisions and work as a team to resolve the problem.

6. Emergency simulation :
- Nurses regularly take part in emergency simulation sessions to practise managing critical scenarios. This helps them maintain their skills and improve their responsiveness in the event of a crisis.

7. Monitoring and analysis :
- After an emergency situation, the nurses take part in a detailed analysis to assess the team's response, identify strengths and areas for improvement, and make adjustments to protocols if necessary.

Preparation for emergency scenarios is essential to ensure a rapid and effective response in the event of unforeseen complications during surgery. Operating theatre nurses are key members of the healthcare team who play a vital role in managing emergency situations, ensuring the safety and well-being of the patient.

The availability of resources and protocols to respond to critical situations is a crucial aspect of preparation in the operating theatre. Nurses must ensure that all the necessary materials, equipment and protocols are ready to be used should the need arise, in order to guarantee the patient's safety and well-being. Here's how nurses ensure that resources and protocols are available to respond to critical situations:

1. Preoperative check :
- The nurses carry out a thorough check of all the equipment, instruments and resources needed before the start of each operation. This includes emergency trolleys, emergency drugs, resuscitation devices, intubation kits and other equipment specific to the procedure.

2. Maintaining the inventory :
- Nurses manage the inventory of emergency resources and equipment to ensure that they are constantly available, in adequate quantities and in compliance with safety standards.

3. Continuing education :
  - Nurses receive ongoing training in the correct use of emergency equipment and protocols. This ensures that they are competent and confident to react quickly and effectively in critical situations.

4. Regular review of protocols :
  - Nurses participate in regular reviews of emergency protocols with the surgical team. These reviews enable the protocols to be updated in line with current best practice and new medical discoveries.

5. Simulation of critical scenarios :
  - Nurses take part in critical scenario simulations where emergency situations are realistically reproduced. This enables them to put emergency protocols into practice and identify areas for improvement.

6. Communication with suppliers :
  - Nurses maintain communication links with suppliers to ensure that emergency equipment and resources are available in sufficient quantities and meet quality standards.

7. Precise documentation :
  - All audits, training and updates to resources and protocols are carefully documented. This allows progress to be tracked, accurate records to be maintained and compliance to be guaranteed.

The availability of resources and protocols to respond to critical situations is essential to ensure patient safety in the operating theatre. Operating theatre nurses play an essential role in ensuring that emergency equipment is ready for use and that the appropriate protocols are in place to respond effectively when needed.

Patient care and support

Comforting patients and explaining the surgical process to them are fundamental aspects of the role of nurses in the operating theatre. Prior to surgery, patients may experience anxiety, stress and uncertainty. Nurses play a key role in allaying these

47

concerns and helping patients understand what to expect. Here's how nurses comfort patients and explain the surgical process:

1. Creating a reassuring environment :
   - Nurses establish a bond of trust with the patient by creating a warm and reassuring environment. They use empathic communication skills to show that they are there to support the patient throughout the process.

2. Active listening :
   - Nurses listen carefully to the patient's concerns, questions and emotions. They provide a safe space for the patient to express their fears and worries.

3. Explanation of the surgical process :
   - Nurses explain the surgical procedure in simple, understandable terms. They describe the stages, the roles of each member of the surgical team and the objectives of the surgery.

4. Answers to questions :
   - Nurses provide detailed answers to patients' questions about surgery, anaesthesia, the duration of the procedure, potential risks and the recovery process.

5. Use of visual aids :
   - Sometimes nurses use visual aids such as diagrams, explanatory videos or brochures to help patients understand the procedure better.

6. Emotional preparation :
   - Nurses help patients prepare emotionally by addressing the physical and emotional aspects of surgery. They discuss the normal emotions the patient may experience and offer strategies for coping with anxiety.

7. Support :
   - The nurses remain at the patient's side throughout the pre-operative process, providing constant and encouraging support.

8. Coordination with the surgical team :
- Nurses communicate the patient's concerns and needs to the surgical team to ensure that the patient receives the necessary support and information.

Reassurance and explanation of the surgical process play an essential role in the patient's mental and emotional preparation. Operating theatre nurses are invaluable support workers who help patients feel confident, informed and ready for the surgery ahead.

Emotional and mental preparation for surgery is an important step for patients before an operation. Operating theatre nurses play a key role in helping patients cope with anxiety, manage their emotions and prepare mentally for the procedure. Here's how nurses help prepare patients emotionally and mentally for surgery:

1. Validation of emotions :
- Nurses validate the patient's emotions by recognising and normalising feelings of anxiety, fear or uncertainty. They show empathy and provide a space for the patient to express their concerns.

2. Information and education :
- Nurses provide precise information about the surgical procedure, the steps involved, the risks and the benefits. They help the patient understand what to expect, which can reduce uncertainty and anxiety.

3. Relaxation techniques :
- Nurses teach patients relaxation techniques such as deep breathing, positive visualisation and meditation. These techniques help to ease anxiety and promote relaxation.

4. Stress management :
- Nurses offer advice on stress management, including advice on time management, relaxation exercises and activities that promote well-being.

5. Physical preparation :
- The nurses help the patient to prepare physically by explaining the pre-operative measures, such as fasting and

personal hygiene, which are essential for safety during surgery.

6. Discussion of concerns :
   - The nurses listen to the patient's specific concerns about the surgery, the risks, recovery, etc. They answer questions thoroughly to allay any concerns.

7. Emotional support :
   - Nurses provide constant emotional support by encouraging the patient, offering reassuring words and being present to meet psychological needs.

8. Working with the care team :
   - Nurses work with psychologists, social workers or other mental health professionals to provide comprehensive support to patients with specific emotional needs.

Emotional and mental preparation for surgery can help to reduce anxiety, improve pain tolerance and promote a faster recovery. Operating theatre nurses are essential members of the health care team who offer valuable support to help patients approach surgery with confidence and serenity.

Interdisciplinary communication

Coordination with the surgical team, comprising surgeons, anaesthetists, nurses and operating theatre assistants, is essential to ensure that surgical procedures run smoothly and safely. Operating theatre nurses play a key role in this coordination by facilitating communication and ensuring that each member of the team works in a harmonious and coordinated manner. Here's how nurses coordinate with the various members of the surgical team:

1. Surgeons :
   - Operating room nurses work closely with surgeons by providing logistical support, preparing the operating room with the necessary instruments and equipment, and anticipating the surgeon's specific needs during the procedure.

2. Anaesthetists :

- Nurses work closely with anaesthetists to prepare the patient for anaesthesia, monitor vital signs during induction and ensure patient safety throughout the procedure.

3. Nurses and operating theatre assistants :

- Operating room nurses work as a team with other nurses and operating room assistants to prepare the operating room, ensure workflow during surgery, supply the surgeons with the necessary instruments and constantly monitor the patient's needs.

4. Ongoing communication :

- Nurses facilitate ongoing communication between members of the surgical team by passing on important information, relaying concerns and sharing updates on the patient's condition.

5. Emergency management :

- In the event of an emergency or complication during surgery, the nurses coordinate with the surgical team to take rapid and appropriate action to ensure the patient's safety.

6. Respect for roles and responsibilities :

- Operating room nurses respect the roles and responsibilities of each member of the surgical team, contributing to a collaborative and harmonious working environment.

7. Postoperative revision :

- After surgery, the nurses coordinate with the team to ensure that the patient is stable, safely transferred and that post-operative procedures are in place.

Effective coordination with the surgical team is essential to ensure high quality surgical care and patient safety. Operating theatre nurses play a central role in facilitating communication, anticipating needs and ensuring that each member of the team works together to achieve the best possible outcome for the patient.

Effective information exchange is a cornerstone of safe and smooth surgery in the operating theatre. Nurses play an essential role in the smooth and accurate transmission of information between members of the surgical team to ensure optimum coordination and minimise risks. Here's how nurses facilitate the exchange of information to ensure safe and smooth surgery:

1. Preoperative briefing :
   • Before the surgery begins, the nurses organise a pre-operative briefing during which the members of the surgical team discuss the details of the procedure, the patient's allergies, potential risks and any other relevant information.

2. Using the SBAR method :
   • Nurses frequently use the SBAR method (Situation, Background, Assessment, Recommendation) to structure important communications. This ensures that information is conveyed clearly and concisely.

3. Verbal communication :
   • Nurses communicate verbally with surgeons, anaesthetists, nurses and operating theatre assistants during surgery to share updates on the patient's condition, the progress of the procedure and specific needs.

4. Use of communication tools :
   • Nurses use communication tools such as whiteboards, e-mail systems and radios to transmit important information in real time.

5. Changes to the care plan :
   • If adjustments need to be made to the care plan or surgical procedure, the nurses quickly communicate these changes to the team to ensure that everyone is informed and in agreement.

6. Transfer ratio :
   • At the end of surgery, the nurses prepare a detailed transfer report for post-operative care. They pass on information about the procedure, the medicines

administered, the patient's reactions and any other relevant information.

7. Postoperative debriefing :
- After surgery, the nurses organise a post-operative debriefing to discuss events during the surgery, identify positive points and areas for improvement, and share lessons learned.

8. Compliance with confidentiality protocols :
- Nurses ensure that information shared complies with confidentiality and patient data protection protocols.

A clear, complete and timely exchange of information is essential for patient safety and the success of surgery. Operating theatre nurses are communication facilitators who ensure that every member of the surgical team is informed and involved, contributing to informed decision-making and effective co-ordination of care.

Personal preparation and well-being

Managing stress and anxiety prior to surgery is a crucial aspect of the operating theatre nurse's role. Patients may experience a range of negative emotions prior to surgery, including anxiety, fear and uncertainty. Nurses play a vital role in helping patients manage these emotions to promote a positive state of mind and contribute to optimal surgical outcomes. Here's how nurses manage patients' stress and anxiety before surgery:

1. Empathetic communication :
- Nurses actively listen to patients' concerns and fears with empathy. They show that they understand the patient's emotions and provide a space for them to express themselves.

2. Education and information :
- Nurses provide detailed information about the surgical procedure, the stages, risks, benefits and recovery process. A clear understanding can reduce the anxiety associated with the unknown.

3. Relaxation techniques :
   - Nurses teach patients relaxation techniques such as deep breathing, visualisation and meditation to help calm the mind and reduce stress.

4. Expectation management :
   - Nurses discuss realistic expectations of the surgery and the postoperative period with patients, which can help to reduce undue apprehension.

5. Encouragement to ask questions :
   - Nurses encourage patients to ask questions and express their concerns. This allows patients to feel better informed and more in control.

6. Emotional support :
   - Nurses offer emotional support by providing encouragement, reassurance and being there for patients' emotional needs.

7. Distraction :
   - Nurses can use distraction techniques, such as soothing music or light conversation, to help patients relax before surgery.

8. Collaboration with mental health professionals :
   - Nurses work with psychologists or social workers to offer additional psychological support to patients with high levels of stress or anxiety.

Managing stress and anxiety before surgery is an essential part of pre-operative care. Operating theatre nurses play a key role in providing emotional support, clear information and strategies to help patients approach surgery with greater calm and confidence, which can have a positive impact on their overall experience and recovery.

Self-care techniques are essential for operating theatre nurses to maintain concentration, alertness and well-being during demanding surgical procedures. Working in a stressful and demanding environment can have an impact on performance and mental health. Here's how nurses use self-care techniques to maintain their concentration and alertness:

1. Stress management :
   - Nurses use stress management techniques such as meditation, yoga, deep breathing and muscle relaxation to reduce stress and promote mental clarity.

2. Break and recovery :
   - Nurses regularly take breaks to rest and recharge their batteries. A short break can help maintain concentration throughout the day.

3. A balanced diet :
   - A healthy, balanced diet provides nurses with the energy they need to remain alert. Avoiding heavy meals before surgery can also prevent drowsiness.

4. Adequate hydration :
   - Drinking enough water throughout the day can help prevent dehydration, which can affect concentration and performance.

5. Quality sleep :
   - Nurses strive to get adequate, quality sleep to maintain their alertness during the long hours they work in the operating theatre.

6. Physical exercise :
   - Regular exercise helps to improve blood circulation, boost energy levels and stimulate concentration.

7. Time management :
   - Planning and organising tasks effectively can reduce stress and help nurses stay focused on their responsibilities.
8. Use of soothing music :
   - Listening to soothing music during breaks or moments of relaxation can help reduce stress and promote concentration.

9. Social support :
   - Support and positive interaction with colleagues can help maintain morale and reduce stress.

10. Professional development :
Taking part in ongoing training and learning sessions can help nurses feel more competent and confident in their role, which can reduce stress and improve concentration.

By adopting self-care techniques, operating theatre nurses are better equipped to maintain their concentration, alertness and well-being while providing high-quality patient care. These practices also promote resilience and help prevent burnout.

Chapter 3:
Sterilisation and asepsis techniques

The importance of sterilisation and asepsis in the operating theatre

The importance of sterilisation and asepsis in the operating theatre cannot be overstated. These practices are essential to prevent nosocomial infections, reduce post-operative complications and ensure patient safety during and after surgery. Operating theatre nurses play a vital role in implementing and maintaining high standards of sterilisation and asepsis. Here's why these measures are so crucial:

1. Infection prevention :
   • Sterilisation and asepsis are the cornerstones of healthcare-associated infection (HAI) prevention. Minimising the presence of pathogenic micro-organisms in the surgical environment considerably reduces the risk of infection in patients made vulnerable by surgery.

2. Minimisation of post-operative complications :
   • Post-operative infections can lead to serious complications, delay recovery and prolong hospital stays. By maintaining rigorous sterilisation and asepsis practices, nurses help to minimise these risks.

3. Guaranteeing patient safety :
   • Infections linked to poor sterilisation or a lack of asepsis can be life-threatening. Nurses have a responsibility to create a safe surgical environment by following strict protocols.

4. Compliance with regulatory standards :
   • Hospitals and clinics are subject to strict infection control regulations. Operating theatre nurses must meet these standards to comply with legal and ethical requirements.

5. Promoting patient confidence :
- Patients expect to receive safe, high-quality care. Effective implementation of sterilisation and asepsis reinforces patient confidence in the healthcare system and in the surgical team.

6. Improved surgical results :
- By reducing infections and complications, operating theatre nurses help to improve the overall outcomes of surgical procedures, resulting in faster recovery and shorter hospital stays.

7. Preserving the efficacy of antibiotics :
- Excessive use of antibiotics can lead to drug resistance. Sterilisation and asepsis reduce the need for postoperative antibiotic therapy, helping to preserve the effectiveness of antibiotics.

In short, sterilisation and asepsis are fundamental pillars of safety and quality of care in the operating theatre. Operating theatre nurses play a vital role in ensuring that these high standards are maintained at all times, contributing directly to the safety, health and recovery of patients.

Operating theatre nurses play a critical role in preventing hospital-acquired infections, also known as healthcare-associated infections (HAIs). Their commitment to rigorous infection control practices is essential to ensure patient safety and recovery. Here's how nurses play a key role in preventing hospital-acquired infections in the operating theatre:

1. Application of sterilisation and asepsis protocols :
- Nurses are responsible for the strict implementation of sterilisation and asepsis protocols to prevent microbial contamination during surgery. They ensure that all instruments, equipment and the environment are properly sterilised to prevent the introduction of pathogens.

2. Monitoring hygiene procedures :
- Nurses constantly monitor hygiene procedures, ensuring that all members of the surgical team wear appropriate clothing, wash their hands properly and use personal protective equipment (PPE) in accordance with standards.

3. Preventing cross-contamination :
  • Nurses ensure that surfaces, instruments and supplies are kept in sterile areas and avoid cross-contamination between patients. They also supervise the proper placement of sterile drapes to isolate the operating area.

4. Management of medical devices :
  • Nurses properly manage medical devices, such as catheters and drains, to minimise the risk of infection. They ensure that devices are inserted and handled according to best practice.

5. Patient monitoring :
  • Nurses constantly monitor the patient's vital signs and general condition during surgery, enabling them to detect any signs of potential infection at an early stage.

6. Prevention of post-operative complications :
  • Nurses monitor patients closely after surgery, making sure dressings are kept clean and dry, and watching for signs of infection. Early detection and rapid intervention can prevent post-operative complications.

7. Patient education :
  • Nurses educate patients on postoperative hygiene measures and the signs of infection to look out for after discharge from hospital.

8. Interdisciplinary communication :
  • Nurses work closely with other members of the care team, such as surgeons, anaesthetists and intensive care nurses, to share important information about the patient's condition and infection management.

The role of operating theatre nurses in preventing hospital-acquired infections is fundamental to ensuring the safety and quality of care. Their vigilance, expertise and commitment to best practice in infection control are crucial to minimising risk and contributing to positive outcomes for patients.

Post-operative infections have serious and potentially fatal consequences for patients. These infections occur after surgery and can be associated with complications that affect the patient's recovery. Operating theatre nurses play a crucial role in preventing these infections to minimise the harmful consequences. Here are some of the consequences of post-operative infections for patients:

1. Extended hospital stay :
   - Post-operation infections can lead to a longer hospital stay. Patients have to undergo additional observation and treatment, which can delay their recovery and increase healthcare costs.

2. Increased pain and discomfort :
   - Infections can cause increased pain and discomfort for patients already weakened by surgery. This can compromise their quality of life during the recovery period.

3. Delayed recovery :
   - Infections often delay the healing process. Patients may need more time to recover and regain their strength after a post-operative infection.

4. Additional complications :
   - Infections can lead to other medical complications, such as abscesses, septicaemia (blood infections) or internal organ infections, which can worsen the patient's condition.

5. Increased risk of rehospitalisation :
   - Patients with a post-operative infection are more likely to be readmitted to hospital for further treatment, placing emotional and financial burdens on them and their families.

6. Impact on long-term quality of life :
   - Serious post-operative infections can have a lasting impact on patients' quality of life, affecting their ability to function normally and resume their daily activities.

7. Rising healthcare costs :
   - The additional treatments required to treat post-operative infections result in additional healthcare costs for patients and healthcare systems.

8. Mortality risk :
- In serious cases, post-operative infections can lead to an increased risk of death, particularly in patients already weakened by surgery.

Operating theatre nurses play a major role in preventing post-operative infections by ensuring that the environment is properly sterilised, that hygiene protocols are followed, that vital signs are constantly monitored and that preventive measures are implemented. By minimising the risk of infection, nurses contribute directly to the safety, recovery and quality of care for surgical patients.

Fundamental principles of sterilisation

Understanding the different types of sterilisation is essential for operating theatre nurses to ensure patient safety and infection prevention. Each sterilisation method aims to eliminate or kill pathogenic micro-organisms present on surgical instruments, equipment and surfaces. Here's an overview of the different types of sterilisation that nurses need to know about:

1. Steam sterilisation (autoclave) :
- Steam sterilisation is one of the most common methods used in operating theatres. It uses moist heat in the form of saturated steam to destroy micro-organisms. Nurses must follow precise protocols to load, run and unload autoclaves correctly.

2. Gas sterilisation (ethylene oxide) :
- Ethylene oxide gas is used to sterilise materials that are sensitive to heat and moisture, such as electronic instruments or plastic materials. Nurses should be aware of the handling, degassing and ventilation protocols associated with this method.

3. Sterilisation by radiation (gamma rays, X-rays) :
- Ionising radiation, such as gamma rays and X-rays, is used to destroy micro-organisms by damaging their DNA. This method is often used to sterilise medical materials that are sensitive to heat and humidity.

4. Chemical sterilisation :
- Certain chemicals, such as glutaraldehyde, can be used for the cold sterilisation of certain instruments and equipment. Nurses must follow specific protocols to dilute chemicals correctly and ensure effective sterilisation.

5. Sterilisation by filtration :
- Filtration sterilisation uses special filters to eliminate micro-organisms from liquids or gases. This can be used to sterilise medical solutions or respiratory gases.

6. Plasma sterilisation :
- Plasma sterilisation uses an ionised gas to destroy micro-organisms. It is a gentle method that can be used for materials sensitive to heat and humidity.

7. Dry heat sterilisation :
- Dry heat sterilisation uses hot air to destroy micro-organisms. It is less common than steam sterilisation, but can be used for certain types of material.

Operating theatre nurses must understand the benefits, limitations and protocols associated with each sterilisation method. They are responsible for ensuring that instruments, equipment and surfaces are correctly sterilised before each surgical procedure to prevent nosocomial infections and ensure patient safety.

Validation and monitoring of sterilisation cycles are essential elements of the operating theatre nurse's role in ensuring the effectiveness of sterilisation procedures. The aim of these activities is to check that the sterilisation methods used have achieved the objectives of destroying pathogenic micro-organisms and maintaining high standards of patient safety. Here's how nurses validate and monitor sterilisation cycles:

1. Checking the parameters :
- The nurses regularly check the sterilisation parameters, such as temperature, pressure, time and humidity, to ensure that they comply with the standards set by the equipment manufacturers and the establishment's protocols.

2. Use of biological indicators :
   - Nurses use biological indicators, such as bacterial spores, to assess the effectiveness of sterilisation. These spores are placed in control loads and tested after the sterilisation cycle to confirm that the micro-organisms have been destroyed.

3. Chemical controls :
   - Nurses use chemical indicators to monitor sterilisation cycles. Chemical indicators change colour according to exposure to specific conditions, helping to confirm that cycles have been carried out correctly.

4. Initial validation :
   - Before using a new sterilisation method or piece of equipment, nurses carry out an initial validation to ensure that the sterilisation parameters specified by the manufacturer are achieved and that efficacy is proven.

5. Load tests :
   - Nurses carry out load tests by placing control loads in the sterilisation cycles. These control loads contain specific items and are analysed to check the effectiveness of the sterilisation.

6. Precise documentation :
   - Nurses carefully document the details of each sterilisation cycle, including parameters, indicators used and test results. Accurate documentation is essential for monitoring and ensuring compliance with sterilisation standards.

7. Further training :
   - Nurses undergo continuous training to keep up to date with the latest sterilisation practices and techniques, helping them to maintain their expertise in this critical area.

Validation and monitoring of sterilisation cycles are essential steps in ensuring patient safety in the operating theatre. Operating theatre nurses play a key role in ensuring that instruments and equipment are correctly sterilised, which contributes directly to the prevention of nosocomial infections and to patient safety.

Preparation and packaging of sterile materials

Packaging techniques play a crucial role in maintaining the sterility integrity of surgical instruments and equipment after sterilisation. Improper handling or use of packaging materials can compromise sterility and increase the risk of post-operative infections. Operating theatre nurses need to master different packaging techniques to ensure that items remain sterile until they are used. These include

1. Use of appropriate packaging materials :
   - Nurses should select appropriate packaging materials according to the type of instruments and equipment to be sterilised. Packaging must be heat, moisture and puncture resistant to prevent contamination.

2. Double envelope technique :
   - Double-wrap packaging involves wrapping instruments in a first layer of packaging, then placing them in a second layer. This creates an additional barrier against contamination.

3. Appropriate folding technique :
   - Nurses must learn appropriate folding techniques to avoid folds or air pockets in the packaging, as these could become havens for micro-organisms.

4. Use of chemical indicators :
   - Nurses can insert chemical indicators inside the pack to visually check whether sterilisation has been achieved. This allows them to quickly identify any packaging that may have been compromised during the process.

5. Use of indicator tapes :
   - The self-adhesive indicator tapes change colour when the required sterilisation parameters have been reached. They provide visual confirmation that instruments have been correctly sterilised.

6. Compliance with handling protocols :
   - Nurses must follow strict protocols when handling packaged sterile items. This includes rules on where items can be opened and how they should be handled to avoid contamination.

7. Marking and labelling :
- Packaged packs should be clearly marked and labelled with information such as the sterilisation date, the contents and the name of the operator. This facilitates tracking and rapid identification of the contents.

8. Appropriate storage :
- Packaged packs should be stored in a clean, dry environment to avoid any risk of contamination before use.

Mastery of packaging techniques is essential to maintaining the sterile integrity of instruments and equipment in the operating theatre. Nurses play a crucial role in this process by ensuring that instruments are correctly packaged, handled and stored, which contributes directly to the prevention of nosocomial infections and to patient safety.

The use of protective barriers and safety devices is essential practice in the operating theatre to minimise the risks of cross-contamination, exposure to body fluids and sharp instrument accidents. Operating theatre nurses play a central role in the implementation and use of these protective measures to ensure the safety of patients, the surgical team and themselves. Here are some examples of the use of protective barriers and safety devices:

1. Sterile gloves :
- Operating theatre nurses wear sterile gloves to avoid direct contact with surfaces, instruments and patients, thereby reducing the risk of cross-contamination. Gloves must be changed regularly and correctly according to the needs of the procedure.

2. Gowns and masks :
- Sterile gowns and masks are worn to prevent contamination of instruments and the environment by hair, skin particles and respiratory droplets. This also helps prevent the transmission of pathogens from the surgical team to the patient.

3. Protective goggles and face shields :
   - To minimise the risk of exposure to splashes of body fluids, nurses can wear protective goggles or face shields during potentially risky procedures.

4. Use of sterile drapes :
   - Sterile drapes are special blankets made of sterile fabric that are used to isolate the operating area and create a barrier between the patient and the rest of the environment. Nurses ensure that the drapes are correctly positioned to maintain sterility.

5. Safety devices for sharp instruments :
   - Nurses use sharp instruments fitted with safety devices, such as safety needles, to reduce the risk of exposure to puncture wounds.

6. Appropriate management of biomedical waste :
   - Nurses ensure that biomedical waste, such as contaminated instruments and disposable materials, are disposed of in accordance with safety protocols to prevent the spread of infection.

7. Preventing exposure to radiation :
   - During radiological procedures in the operating theatre, nurses use lead aprons and other protective equipment to minimise exposure to ionising radiation.

8. Protection against chemicals :
   - When using chemicals, nurses wear appropriate personal protective equipment to minimise the risk of skin or respiratory exposure.

The appropriate use of protective barriers and safety devices is crucial to maintaining a safe and sterile environment in the operating theatre. Operating theatre nurses must be trained in the correct use of these protective measures and be vigilant in their application to prevent accidents, minimise the risk of contamination and ensure the safety of all members of the surgical team and patients.

Sterilisation of surgical instruments

The process of cleaning, disinfecting and sterilising surgical instruments is a critical step in preventing nosocomial infections and ensuring patient safety in the operating theatre. Operating theatre nurses play a central role in these processes to ensure that the instruments used during surgery are clean, disinfected and sterile. The following are the stages in the process of cleaning, disinfecting and sterilising instruments:

1. Pre-cleaning :
   - Immediately after the end of the surgical procedure, the instruments are pre-cleaned to remove biological tissue, body fluids and any other visible material. This is usually done using warm water and an enzymatic detergent. Nurses take care not to allow debris to dry on the instruments.

2. Visual inspection :
   - Pre-cleaned instruments are visually inspected to ensure that they are clean and that all visible debris has been removed. If contaminants remain, the instruments undergo another pre-cleaning cycle.

3. Mechanical or manual cleaning :
   - The instruments undergo a more thorough cleaning using mechanical (washer-disinfector) or manual methods. The aim is to eliminate any remaining organic residues. Nurses follow the facility's protocols to ensure thorough cleaning.

4. Rinsing :
   - After cleaning, the instruments are thoroughly rinsed to remove detergent residues and contaminants.

5. Disinfection :
   - Some instruments, even though they have been cleaned, require an additional disinfection step to kill any remaining micro-organisms. Nurses use appropriate chemical disinfectants, following the manufacturer's instructions.

6. Final rinse :
   - Disinfected instruments are carefully rinsed again to remove any disinfectant residue.

7. Drying :
  • The instruments are carefully dried to prevent bacterial growth due to humidity.

8. Final inspection :
  • Before sterilisation, the instruments are visually inspected again to ensure that they are clean and in good condition.

9. Sterilisation :
  • Instruments are subjected to an appropriate sterilisation process, such as steam, gas, radiation, etc., depending on the type of instrument and the established protocols.

10. Sterility check :
  • After sterilisation, the instruments are checked using chemical or biological indicators to confirm that the sterilisation process has been successful.

11. Storage :
  • Sterile instruments are stored in sterile packs until they are used in the operating theatre.

Operating theatre nurses must rigorously follow these steps to ensure that surgical instruments are clean, disinfected and sterile before each operation. Their expertise in the cleaning, disinfection and sterilisation process contributes directly to the prevention of nosocomial infections and to patient safety.

The use of autoclaves and other sterilisation devices in the hospital environment is a crucial practice for ensuring patient safety by preventing the transmission of nosocomial infections. Operating theatre nurses play an essential role in operating and monitoring these devices to ensure the sterility of medical instruments and equipment. Here's how nurses use autoclaves and other sterilisation devices in the hospital environment:

1. Autoclaves :
  • Autoclaves are devices that use moist heat in the form of saturated steam to sterilise instruments and equipment. Nurses load instruments into special trays, follow the appropriate loading protocols and select the sterilisation parameters (temperature, pressure, time) according to the type of instrument and material. They monitor the process

to ensure that the parameters are met and that sterilisation is successful.

2. Gas sterilisers :
   • Gas sterilisers use chemical gases, such as ethylene oxide, to sterilise instruments and equipment that are sensitive to heat and humidity. Nurses place the items to be sterilised in special chambers and follow safety protocols for handling the gas and degassing the items after sterilisation.

3. Radiation sterilisation :
   • Radiation sterilisers, such as gamma sterilisers, use ionising radiation to destroy micro-organisms. Nurses place the items in special containers and send them to an external sterilisation facility.

4. Plasma sterilisation :
   • Plasma sterilisers use an ionised gas to sterilise instruments. Nurses place items in special chambers and follow protocols for exposing items to plasma.

5. Monitoring and documentation :
   • Nurses carefully monitor sterilisation cycles, using chemical and biological indicators to check the effectiveness of sterilisation. They carefully document each cycle, recording parameters, test results and details of the instruments sterilised.

6. Device maintenance :
   • Nurses carry out regular maintenance on autoclaves and other sterilisation equipment to ensure that they are working properly. They ensure that the devices are calibrated correctly and that all parts are in good condition.

7. Further training :
   • Nurses undergo continuous training to keep up to date with the latest sterilisation practices and techniques, helping them to maintain their expertise in this crucial area.

The proper use of autoclaves and other sterilisation equipment is essential to prevent nosocomial infections and ensure patient safety. Operating theatre nurses play a key role in this process by ensuring that instruments and equipment are correctly sterilised, which contributes directly to the quality of care and patient safety.

Aseptic techniques for the operating theatre

Personal hygiene habits and the wearing of appropriate clothing are essential aspects of the professional practice of operating theatre nurses. These measures help to maintain a sterile environment, prevent the spread of infections and ensure the safety of patients and the surgical team. Here's how operating theatre nurses approach these aspects:

1. Shower and personal hygiene :
   - Operating theatre nurses follow strict personal hygiene practices. They take a shower before starting their shift to eliminate body contaminants and micro-organisms. Special care is taken to keep hair, nails and skin clean.

2. Hand washing :
   - Hand washing is one of the most fundamental hygiene habits. Operating theatre nurses wash their hands thoroughly with antiseptic soap before and after each operation, as well as at any time when contamination is possible.

3. Wear suitable clothing :
   - Nurses wear specific clothing in the operating theatre to minimise contamination. This includes sterile gowns, trousers, shoe covers and caps. Personal clothing is kept outside the operating theatre.

4. Use of masks and eye protection :
   - Nurses wear face masks and goggles to prevent respiratory droplets and splashes of body fluids from contaminating the operating area.

5. Preparation in surgical garb :
   - Operating theatre nurses prepare by wearing special surgical attire, including sterile gloves, before entering the operating theatre. They ensure that each piece of equipment is correctly fitted.

6. Regular change of gloves and gowns:
- Operating theatre nurses regularly change their gloves and gowns to prevent cross-contamination and maintain sterility.

7. Avoidance of risky behaviour :
- Operating room nurses avoid touching non-sterile surfaces or their faces during procedures. They refrain from chewing gum, drinking, eating or handling their mobile phones during surgery.

8. Attitude of constant vigilance :
- Nurses maintain a vigilant attitude to personal hygiene, being aware of their actions and movements to avoid contamination.

These personal hygiene habits and the wearing of appropriate clothing are essential for creating and maintaining a sterile environment in the operating theatre. Nurses play a key role in promoting these practices to ensure patient safety and prevent nosocomial infections.

Hand-washing practices and the use of disinfectants are an integral part of strict hygiene measures in the operating theatre. Operating theatre nurses are required to follow specific protocols to ensure that their hands are clean and free from contaminants before and during surgical procedures. Here's how nurses approach hand-washing practices and the use of disinfectants:

1. Washing hands before surgery :
- Before entering the operating theatre, nurses wash their hands thoroughly with antiseptic soap. They make sure to wash all parts of their hands, including the fingernails and interdigital spaces.

2. Surgical hand washing :
- Before setting up the sterile operating area, nurses perform a thorough surgical hand wash. This process involves several stages of washing, rinsing and drying to ensure maximum cleanliness.

3. Use of alcohol-based disinfectants :
   - Operating theatre nurses regularly use alcohol-based disinfectants to reduce the proliferation of micro-organisms on the hands. This can be done between hand washes to maintain sterility.

4. Hand washing between tasks :
   - Nurses wash their hands systematically between different tasks, such as handling sterile and non-sterile instruments, to avoid cross-contamination.

5. Wearing gloves :
   - Gloves are worn in addition to hand washing to create an extra protective barrier. However, hand washing remains essential, as gloves do not guarantee complete protection.

6. Avoiding contamination during operations :
   - During surgery, nurses avoid touching non-sterile surfaces or their faces. If gloves are contaminated, they change them immediately and wash their hands.

7. Aseptic practices :
   - Nurses follow rigorous aseptic practices, including hand-washing protocols, when preparing sterile instruments for surgery.

8. Further training :
   - Operating theatre nurses undergo continuous training in the latest hygiene practices and the use of disinfectants to keep up to date and maintain high standards of hygiene.

The strict application of hand-washing practices and the use of disinfectants are crucial in reducing the risk of contamination and preventing nosocomial infections in the operating theatre. Nurses play a fundamental role in implementing these measures to guarantee patient safety and maintain a sterile environment during surgery.

Maintaining asepsis during surgery

The use of sterile drapes and barriers in the operating theatre is an essential practice to prevent cross-contamination and maintain a sterile environment during surgical procedures.

Operating theatre nurses play a key role in setting up and maintaining these barriers to ensure patient safety and the success of surgical procedures. Here's how nurses use sterile drapes and barriers to prevent contamination:

1. Use of sterile drapes :
   • Sterile drapes are special blankets made of sterile fabric used to isolate the operating area and prevent contamination from outside. Operating theatre nurses ensure that drapes are correctly positioned to cover the area where surgery will take place. This includes creating a sterile opening the size of the surgical drape, through which the surgeons work.

2. Creation of sterile and non-sterile zones :
   • Nurses clearly mark and demarcate sterile and non-sterile areas using sterile drapes, sheets, adhesive tape or other methods. Instruments and surgical teams remain in the sterile zone, while staff outside the sterile zone avoid contact with sterile objects.

3. Handling sterile drapes :
   • Nurses handle sterile drapes with care to avoid contaminating them. They wear sterile gloves and use sterile forceps to handle the drapes, avoiding any contact with non-sterile surfaces.

4. Barriers for instruments and equipment :
   • Instruments and equipment that come into contact with the operating area are covered with sterile drapes to keep them sterile. Nurses ensure that instruments are placed on sterile trays and handled with sterile forceps to avoid contamination.
5. Barriers for team members :
   • Members of the surgical team wear sterile gowns, sterile gloves and masks to prevent contamination. Operating theatre nurses constantly monitor compliance with these barrier measures.

6. Preventing contamination of non-sterile objects :
   • Operating theatre nurses ensure that non-sterile items, such as keys, pens and mobile phones, are kept outside the sterile area to avoid contamination.

7. Monitoring and readjustment :
- Nurses constantly monitor sterile drapes and barriers to ensure that they are not compromised. If sterility is breached, they take immediate action to rectify the situation.

The use of sterile drapes and barriers is fundamental to maintaining a sterile environment in the operating theatre. Nurses play a crucial role in setting up and maintaining these barriers to prevent cross-contamination, reduce the risk of infection and ensure the safety of patients and the surgical team.

Techniques for handling instruments and supplies while maintaining asepsis are essential in the operating theatre to avoid cross-contamination and maintain a sterile environment. Operating theatre nurses follow strict protocols for the careful handling of instruments and supplies during surgical procedures. Here's how they maintain asepsis during handling:

1. Use of sterile forceps and instruments :
- Nurses use sterile tongs to handle instruments and supplies. Sterile tongs allow them to grasp and move objects without directly touching surfaces, minimising the risk of contamination.

  -

2. Handling techniques :
- Operating theatre nurses are trained in specific techniques for handling instruments and supplies aseptically. This may include precise movements to avoid non-sterile contact.

3. Avoid sudden movements :
- Nurses avoid sudden gestures or rapid movements that could generate potentially contaminating droplets or particles.

4. Conscious handling :
- Nurses maintain constant awareness of their movements and the location of instruments and supplies to avoid accidental contamination.

5. Use of sterile drapes as guides :
   - Sterile drapes are used as visual guides to delimit the sterile zone. Nurses handle instruments within these fields and avoid exceeding the sterile limits.

6. Careful preparation of instruments :
   - Before the operation, the nurses carefully prepare the necessary instruments and supplies, ensuring that they are correctly arranged and ready to be used without compromising asepsis.

7. Using wizards :
   - Nurses may work with other members of the surgical team to transfer instruments aseptically, using sterile forceps or other approved methods.

8. Avoid excessive movement:
   - Nurses avoid excessive movements that could lead to non-sterile contact with other team members or non-sterile objects.

9. Reducing distractions :
   - During operations, nurses concentrate on their tasks and minimise distractions to avoid any situation that could compromise asepsis.

Aseptic handling of instruments and supplies is fundamental to ensuring sterility in the operating theatre. Operating theatre nurses are trained in these techniques and must maintain constant vigilance to avoid cross-contamination and safeguard the safety of patients and the surgical team.

Management of contamination incidents

Operating theatre nurses must be prepared to react quickly and effectively when asepsis is compromised, in order to minimise the risk of contamination and preserve the safety of patients and the surgical team. Here's how they follow protocols to deal with situations where asepsis is compromised:

1. Quick recognition :
   - Nurses must be vigilant and able to immediately recognise any situation where asepsis could be compromised. This

may include inappropriate gestures, non-sterile contact or uncontrolled movements.

2. Immediate communication :
   - As soon as a compromised asepsis situation is identified, nurses must immediately inform members of the surgical team, including surgeons, anaesthetists and other nurses.

3. Insulation and repair :
   - If asepsis is compromised, nurses work closely with the team to isolate the affected area and implement corrective measures. This may include repeating aseptic steps, replacing sterile drapes or rapidly sterilising additional instruments if necessary.

4. Change of gloves and gowns :
   - If asepsis is compromised, nurses immediately change their sterile gloves and gowns to minimise the risk of contamination spreading.

5. Reassessment of the situation :
   - Once corrective measures have been taken, the nurses and surgical team reassess the situation to ensure that asepsis has been re-established before continuing with the operation.

6. Avoid panic:
   - Nurses are trained to remain calm and avoid panic if asepsis is compromised. They work methodically to resolve the problem while maintaining patient safety.

7. Documentation :
   - Any situation where asepsis is compromised must be accurately documented in the patient record. This enables subsequent analysis and continuous improvement of practices.

8. Training and continuing education :
   - Operating theatre nurses undergo regular in-service training to keep abreast of the latest protocols and to maintain their readiness to react quickly if asepsis is compromised.

It is imperative that operating theatre nurses are well trained and prepared to deal with situations where asepsis is compromised. Adherence to appropriate protocols, effective communication within the team and taking immediate corrective action are essential to minimise the risk of contamination and maintain a sterile environment during surgery.

Responding quickly to minimise the risk of infection in the operating theatre is an essential skill for nurses. Their ability to intervene quickly and effectively in risky situations helps to maintain a sterile environment and ensure patient safety. Here's how operating theatre nurses react quickly to minimise the risk of infection:

1. Rapid identification of risks :
   - Nurses are trained to quickly identify potentially risky situations, such as contaminated instruments, inappropriate behaviour or signs of contamination in the operating area.

2. Immediate communication :
   - As soon as a risk of infection is identified, nurses immediately contact members of the surgical team to inform them of the situation. Clear, concise communication is essential if corrective action is to be taken quickly.

3. Insulation and containment :
   - If a potential risk of infection is identified, nurses work with the team to isolate the affected area and prevent the spread of contamination. This may involve closing off non-sterile areas or restricting the team's movements.

4. Impact assessment :
   - Nurses quickly assess the potential impact of the situation on patient safety and the sterility of the environment. This helps them to determine the seriousness of the risk and the action to be taken.

5. Taking corrective action :
   - Nurses take immediate action to correct the risk situation. This may include replacing contaminated instruments, cleaning the affected area or restoring asepsis.

6. Reassessment and monitoring :
  - After taking corrective measures, the nurses reassess the situation to ensure that the risk of infection has been minimised. They carefully monitor the rest of the operation for any potential signs of infection.

7. Precise documentation :
  - All actions taken to minimise the risk of infection must be carefully documented in the patient's file. This enables appropriate follow-up and subsequent analysis of the situation.

8. Further training :
  - Operating theatre nurses take part in ongoing training programmes to enhance their ability to respond quickly and effectively to situations where there is a risk of infection. This keeps them up to date with the latest practices and protocols.

The rapid response of operating theatre nurses is essential to minimising the risk of infection and maintaining patient safety. Their preparation, effective communication within the team and ability to take rapid corrective action all contribute to maintaining a sterile environment and ensuring positive patient outcomes.

Training and updating on best practice

Ongoing training in new sterilisation and asepsis techniques is a crucial component of operating theatre nursing practice. With constant advances in medicine and technology, nurses need to keep up to date with the latest methods and standards to maintain safe and aseptic practices. Here's how continuing education is implemented for new sterilisation and asepsis techniques:

1. Workshops and specialised training :
  - Operating theatre nurses have access to workshops, seminars and specialised training courses focusing on new sterilisation and asepsis techniques. These sessions offer hands-on, interactive learning opportunities, often delivered by leading experts in the field.

2. Online training :
   - E-learning platforms offer a variety of courses and modules on the latest sterilisation and asepsis techniques. Nurses can take these courses at their own pace, to suit their schedule.

3. Medical conferences and congresses :
   - Nurses can attend conferences and medical congresses where the latest advances in sterilisation and asepsis are discussed. These events also provide opportunities for networking with other healthcare professionals.

4. On-site training :
   - Suppliers of medical equipment and sterilisation products can offer on-site training to introduce new technologies and explain their proper use.

5. Protocol updates :
   - Nurses receive regular updates on sterilisation and asepsis protocols and guidelines from regulatory bodies and professional associations. These updates reflect the latest research and best practice.

6. Peer learning :
   - Operating theatre nurses often share their knowledge and experience of sterilisation and asepsis with their colleagues. Exchanges between peers encourage continuous learning and the improvement of skills.

7. Participation in discussion groups :
   - Nurses can take part in online or offline discussion groups, where they can ask questions, share experiences and get advice on new sterilisation and asepsis techniques.

8. Simulation and practical training :
   - Operating theatre simulations and practical training sessions allow nurses to put new sterilisation and asepsis techniques into practice in a controlled environment, encouraging learning by doing.

Ongoing training in new sterilisation and asepsis techniques is fundamental to maintaining the professional competence of operating theatre nurses. It ensures that nurses are well informed about the latest safety standards and the most advanced sterilisation practices, thereby contributing to the prevention of nosocomial infections and to patient safety.

Incorporating national and international guidelines into hospital protocols is a fundamental step in ensuring high-quality, consistent and evidence-based medical practice. Operating theatre nurses play a crucial role in implementing these guidelines to ensure patient safety and well-being. Here's how this integration is achieved:

1. Follow-up of official guidelines :
   - Operating room nurses are responsible for following national and international guidelines issued by bodies such as the World Health Organization (WHO), the Centers for Disease Control and Prevention (CDC) and other government health regulators. They incorporate these guidelines into their protocols to ensure that practice is based on recognised standards.

2. Continuous assessment of practices :
   - Operating room nurses participate in regular evaluations of existing protocols in light of updated guidelines. They identify areas requiring adjustment to comply with current standards.

3. Training and awareness :
   - The nurses are trained in the new guidelines and updated protocols. They then play a key role in making the rest of the surgical team aware of these changes and ensuring that they are properly implemented.

4. Review of hospital protocols :
   - Operating theatre nurses work with other healthcare professionals to review and update hospital protocols, incorporating new guidelines and ensuring that they reflect current best practice.

5. Adherence to quality standards :
   - Nurses ensure that hospital protocols comply with national and international quality standards for patient safety and the prevention of nosocomial infections.

6. Use of best practice :
   - National and international guidelines provide information on best practice in sterilisation, asepsis, patient safety and other critical areas. Nurses incorporate them into their daily practice to optimise surgical outcomes.

7. Reaction to new research :
   - Operating theatre nurses are alert to new research and medical discoveries. When new evidence emerges, they work with the surgical team to assess how these discoveries can be integrated into existing protocols.

8. Professional ethics :
   - By incorporating national and international guidelines into their protocols, nurses demonstrate their commitment to professional ethics and their responsibility to provide high-quality, safe care.

The integration of national and international guidelines into hospital protocols by operating theatre nurses ensures the consistency, safety and quality of surgical care. It reflects their commitment to continuous improvement and helps to ensure positive outcomes for patients.

Monitoring and evaluating the effectiveness of aseptic measures

Regular quality controls are essential in the operating theatre to ensure compliance with sterilisation standards and to maintain a safe and aseptic environment for patients. Operating theatre nurses play a central role in implementing these checks to ensure the safety and well-being of patients. Here's how quality controls are carried out to ensure compliance with sterilisation standards:

1. Visual checks :
   - Nurses carry out regular visual checks to ensure that sterile areas remain intact and that sterile drapes are not compromised. They check that packaging is properly sealed and that instruments and supplies are correctly arranged.

2. Checking expiry dates :
- Nurses regularly check the expiry dates of sterile supplies, disinfectants and sterilisation agents to ensure that they are usable and effective.

3. Sterility tests :
- Nurses can carry out periodic sterility tests on samples of sterile instruments and supplies to check their effectiveness.

4. Checking sterilisation cycles :
- Nurses monitor the sterilisation cycles of autoclaves and other sterilisation devices to ensure that they operate correctly and achieve the required sterilisation parameters.

5. Precise documentation :
- All quality controls and test results are carefully documented. This enables proper monitoring and subsequent analysis to identify trends or potential problems.

6. Further training :
- Nurses take part in ongoing training on best practice in sterilisation and quality control to ensure their competence and understanding of protocols.

7. Working with sterilisation teams :
- The nurses work closely with the sterilisation teams to ensure that the sterilisation processes are followed correctly and that safety standards are met.

8. Incident reports :
- In the event of a problem or non-compliance, nurses quickly report incidents and work with the team to resolve problems and prevent their recurrence.

9. Audits and inspections :
- Operating theatres are regularly audited and inspected to assess compliance with sterilisation standards. Nurses participate in these audits and take corrective action where necessary.

10. Continuous improvement :
- Regular quality controls help to identify areas for improvement. Nurses contribute to the implementation of corrective measures and the continuous improvement of sterilisation practices.

By ensuring compliance with sterilisation standards through rigorous quality controls, operating theatre nurses play a vital role in preventing hospital-acquired infections and ensuring patient safety. Their commitment to quality and safety helps to maintain an aseptic surgical environment and ensure positive patient outcomes.

The use of biological and chemical tests to validate sterility in the operating room is an essential practice to ensure that sterilisation processes have been effective and that instruments and supplies are free from any potentially infectious micro-organisms. Operating theatre nurses play a key role in implementing these tests to ensure patient safety. Here's how biological and chemical tests are used to validate sterility:

1. Biological tests (biological indicators) :
- Nurses use biological indicators to check sterility. These indicators consist of living organisms (usually bacterial spores) which are placed inside the loads to be sterilised. After the sterilisation cycle, these indicators are incubated to determine whether the micro-organisms have been destroyed.

2. Chemical tests (chemical indicators) :
- Chemical indicators, such as strips or stickers, are applied to the packaging of instruments or supplies to be sterilised. They change colour when exposed to specific sterilisation conditions, indicating that the process has been completed.

3. Control of autoclaves :
- Operating theatre nurses monitor autoclaving cycles using biological and chemical indicators. They place the indicators in different areas of the steriliser to ensure that heat and steam have penetrated all parts of the load.

4. Bowie-Dick test :
- This specific test is used to assess steam penetration in autoclave hollow loads. It consists of chemically treated sheets of paper placed in the load and run through a specific sterilisation cycle. Colour changes indicate adequate steam penetration.

5. Enzyme detection tests :
- Some biological indicators contain specific enzymes produced by micro-organisms. Detection of these enzymes after sterilisation indicates the presence of living micro-organisms.

6. Monitoring and documentation :
- The results of all biological and chemical tests are carefully documented. In the event of non-compliance, corrective action is taken, including re-sterilisation if necessary.

7. Training and skills :
- Nurses receive training in the correct use of biological and chemical tests to ensure their competence in performing and interpreting these tests.

8. Incorporating results into protocols :
- The results of biological and chemical tests are taken into account in sterility validation protocols. Nurses work with the surgical team to decide whether sterile loads can be used safely.

The use of biological and chemical tests to validate sterility in the operating theatre is a crucial step in preventing nosocomial infections and ensuring patient safety. Nurses ensure that these tests are correctly performed, documented and interpreted to ensure effective and reliable sterilisation practices.

Chapter 4:
Risk management and safety in the operating theatre

Understanding risks in the operating theatre

Identifying potential risks to patients and the medical team in the operating theatre is a major responsibility for nurses. These professionals play a crucial role in preventing incidents and accidents that could jeopardise the safety and well-being of everyone involved. Here's how nurses identify and manage potential risks:

1. Preoperative assessment :
   - Before each operation, nurses take part in a pre-operative assessment of the patient. They gather information on medical history, allergies, current medication and health problems to identify any potential risks.

2. Checking files :
   - The nurses carefully check the patient's medical records to ensure that all relevant information is taken into account and that the surgical procedures are in line with medical recommendations.

3. Interdisciplinary communication :
   - Nurses interact with members of the surgical team, including surgeons, anaesthetists and operating assistants, to exchange information and identify any potential risks associated with surgery.

4. Anticipating needs :
   - Nurses anticipate the need for equipment, supplies and medicines during surgery to avoid delays and minimise the risks associated with the unavailability of essential resources.
5. Prevention of nosocomial infections :
   - Nurses rigorously apply sterilisation and asepsis protocols to reduce the risk of nosocomial infections and contamination during and after surgery.

6. Managing medication and allergies :
- Nurses check patients for drug allergies and ensure that the medicines administered are appropriate and safe, minimising the risk of intolerance or serious side effects.

7. Emergency preparedness :
- Nurses prepare for emergencies by having the necessary equipment and medicines on hand to manage potential complications.

8. Constant monitoring :
- The nurses constantly monitor the patient's vital signs during the operation to detect any abnormal changes quickly and react accordingly.

9. Postoperative assessment :
- After surgery, nurses monitor patients for any signs of post-operative complications and act quickly to treat them.

10. Analysis of incidents :
- Nurses are involved in analysing incidents and errors to identify the underlying causes and put in place corrective measures to prevent them from happening again.

Identifying potential risks to patients and the medical team is an ongoing and crucial responsibility of operating theatre nurses. Their vigilance, effective communication and commitment to safety help to minimise risks and ensure high-quality surgical care.

Assessing the risk factors associated with specific types of surgery is an essential step in ensuring the safety and success of surgical procedures. Operating theatre nurses play a crucial role in this assessment, working closely with the surgical team to anticipate and mitigate potential risks. Here's how nurses assess risk factors for different types of surgery:

1. Gathering specific information :
- Before each operation, nurses gather specific information about the patient and the procedure. This may include medical history, allergies, current medication and any other relevant factors.

2. Interdisciplinary exchange :
  • Nurses work with the surgical team, including surgeons, anaesthetists and other health professionals, to share information about potential risks associated with surgery.

3. Anticipating complications :
  • Depending on the type of surgery, the nurses anticipate the specific complications that could arise. For example, for cardiac surgery, they focus on close cardiovascular monitoring.

4. Preparing the equipment :
  • Nurses ensure that the equipment needed to manage potential complications is ready and easily accessible.

5. Preventive measures :
  • Nurses implement specific preventive measures depending on the type of surgery. For example, for orthopaedic surgery, they take care to prevent bedsores.

6. Patient assessment :
  • Nurses assess the patient's current condition before surgery to detect any signs of deterioration that could increase the risks.

7. Planning post-operative care :
  • Nurses plan post-operative care taking into account the potential risks associated with surgery. This may include pain management, precautions to avoid pulmonary complications, etc.

8. Close monitoring :
  • During surgery, the nurses constantly monitor the patient's vital signs and react quickly to any abnormal changes.

9. Communication with the patient :
  • Nurses educate patients about the specific risks associated with their surgery and inform them about what they can expect during and after the operation.

10. In-depth documentation :
  • All the risk factors identified, the preventive measures taken and the actions undertaken are carefully documented to ensure traceability and continuity of care.

Assessing the risk factors associated with specific types of surgery is a proactive approach that enables operating room nurses to prepare adequately and take steps to minimise potential risks. Their expertise helps to ensure safer and more successful surgery.

Protocols for the prevention of nosocomial infections

Infection prevention and control measures in the operating theatre are of paramount importance in ensuring an aseptic surgical environment and minimising the risk of nosocomial infections. Operating theatre nurses play a key role in implementing these measures to ensure patient safety. Here's how nurses prevent and control infections in the operating theatre:

1. Sterilisation and asepsis :
   - Nurses ensure that all instruments, supplies and the operating theatre environment are sterile. They strictly follow sterilisation and asepsis protocols to avoid contamination.

2. Hand washing and personal hygiene :
   - Nurses follow strict personal hygiene practices, including thorough hand washing before and after each operation.

3. Wear suitable clothing :
   - Nurses wear specific surgical attire, including gowns, masks, gloves and shoe covers, to minimise the transmission of micro-organisms.

4. Use of sterile drapes :
   - Nurses place sterile drapes around the surgical site to create a protective barrier against contamination.

5. Preparing the patient's skin :
   - Nurses carefully prepare the patient's skin using antiseptics to minimise bacterial colonisation.

6. Air circulation control :
- Nurses maintain controlled air circulation in the operating theatre to reduce the presence of potentially infectious airborne particles.

7. Medical waste management :
- Nurses properly dispose of medical waste, including sharp instruments, biological tissues and contaminated materials, in accordance with safety protocols.

8. Use of sterile equipment :
- Nurses ensure that all equipment used during surgery is sterile and free from contamination.

9. Post-operative precautions :
- After surgery, the nurses ensure that dressings and drains are properly maintained to avoid infections at the surgical site.

10. Monitoring and early detection :
- Nurses constantly monitor post-operative patients for signs of infection and act quickly if any symptoms are suspected.

11. Training and awareness :
- The nurses are trained in infection prevention and control protocols and also make other members of the surgical team aware of the importance of these measures.

By implementing these infection prevention and control measures, operating theatre nurses make a significant contribution to reducing the risk of nosocomial infections and ensuring positive surgical outcomes for patients.

The appropriate use of personal protective equipment (PPE) is essential in the operating theatre to ensure the safety of nurses, the medical team and patients. Nurses must be knowledgeable and skilled in the proper use of PPE to minimise the risk of exposure to infectious agents and potential hazards. Here's how operating theatre nurses use PPE correctly:

1. Masks :
   - Nurses wear surgical masks to prevent the spread of droplets and particles when interacting with the patient or team. Masks must be worn correctly, covering the nose and mouth, and changed regularly.

2. Gloves :
   - Latex or nitrile gloves are worn to protect nurses' hands from body fluids and micro-organisms. Gloves must be put on before any contact with the patient or contaminated equipment, and removed correctly to avoid contamination when they are taken off.

3. Gowns and aprons :
   - Nurses wear sterile gowns or aprons to protect their clothing and prevent cross-contamination. Gowns must be securely fastened and removed correctly to minimise contamination.

4. Overshoes :
   - Shoe covers protect nurses' footwear and prevent contamination of the operating theatre. They must be worn before entering the operating theatre and removed when leaving the sterile area.

5. Protective goggles or face shields :
   - Nurses wear goggles or face shields to protect their eyes and face from potential splashes of fluids during surgery.

6. Surgical helmets :
   - Surgical helmets cover nurses' heads completely to minimise contamination of the sterile environment.

7. Use in layers :
   - Depending on the type of surgery, nurses may need to use several layers of PPE for extra protection.

8. Appropriate removal of PPE :
   - When the surgery is over, the nurses remove the PPE methodically, without contaminating their skin or clothing. They then wash their hands thoroughly.

9. Further training :
  • Nurses receive regular training on the correct use of PPE, including best practice for putting on, adjusting and removing equipment safely.

10. Appropriate disposal :
  • Once used, PPE must be disposed of in accordance with the facility's protocols to avoid any risk of spreading infectious agents.

The appropriate use of PPE in the operating theatre is an essential part of preventing nosocomial infections and ensuring patient safety. Nurses must strictly follow protocols and guidelines to ensure the safe and effective use of PPE.

Emergency preparedness

In the operating theatre, the availability of emergency equipment such as resuscitation trolleys is crucial for responding quickly and effectively to unexpected medical situations that may arise during surgery. Operating theatre nurses play a key role in preparing and managing this emergency equipment to ensure patient safety and the integrity of the medical team. Here's how nurses ensure the availability and appropriate use of this equipment:

1. Preoperative preparation :
  • Before the start of each operation, the nurses check that the resuscitation trolley is properly stocked with essential equipment, such as emergency medicines, ventilation devices, defibrillators, airway management kits, etc.

2. Regular checks :
  • Nurses carry out regular checks to ensure that the resuscitation trolley is complete, in good working order and easily accessible in an emergency.

3. Emergency scenario planning :
  • The nurses anticipate possible emergency scenarios depending on the type of surgery and prepare the resuscitation trolley accordingly.

4. In-depth knowledge of the equipment :
   - Nurses are trained in the correct use of every item on the resuscitation trolley, including drugs, ventilation devices and defibrillators.

5. Quick access :
   - Nurses ensure that the resuscitation trolley is positioned close to the work area and easily accessible at all times.

6. Communication with the team :
   - In the event of an emergency, the nurses quickly inform the surgical team of the availability of the resuscitation trolley and the measures taken.

7. Maintenance and updates :
   - Nurses are responsible for regularly maintaining and updating the equipment on the resuscitation trolley to ensure that it is working properly when needed.

8. Further training :
   - Nurses take part in ongoing training sessions to keep up to date with emergency protocols and the use of resuscitation equipment.

9. Documentation :
   - All actions relating to the use of the resuscitation trolley, including medicines administered and procedures carried out, are carefully documented to ensure complete traceability.

The availability and adequate preparation of emergency equipment, such as resuscitation trolleys, is essential for dealing with critical medical situations in the operating theatre. Operating theatre nurses strive to ensure that this equipment is ready for use when needed, helping to maintain a safe environment and ensure optimal patient care.

Simulating emergency scenarios is an extremely effective teaching method for training operating theatre nurses to react quickly and effectively to critical medical situations. This practical approach enables nurses to develop their crisis management skills, improve their decision-making and boost their confidence in emergency situations. Here's how emergency scenario simulations are conducted for effective operating theatre training:

1. Scenario planning :
   - Trainers devise various emergency scenarios based on realistic medical situations that could arise in the operating theatre, such as cardiac arrest, severe allergic reaction, excessive blood loss, etc.

2. Selection of skills to be assessed :
   - Each scenario is designed to assess specific skills, such as airway management, emergency medication administration, cardiopulmonary resuscitation (CPR), interdisciplinary communication, etc.

3. Setting up the environment :
   - The operating theatre environment is recreated to reflect real-life conditions, with the necessary equipment, instruments and resources close at hand.

4. Scenario implementation :
   - Nurses are placed in simulated emergency situations and have to react as if they were in a real situation. The trainers play the roles of patients, doctors and other team members.

5. Use of high-fidelity mannequins :
   - High-fidelity mannequins, which can simulate vital signs, physiological reactions and responses to interventions, are often used to create more realistic scenarios.

6. Observation and assessment :
   - The trainers carefully observe the nurses' responses and evaluate their actions, decisions and communication during the scenario.

7. Debriefing after simulation :
   - After each scenario, a debriefing session is organised to discuss performance, positive actions and areas for improvement. This allows nurses to learn from their experiences and receive constructive feedback.

8. Continuous learning :
   - Emergency scenario simulations are regularly incorporated into the continuing education programme, enabling nurses

to maintain their skills and familiarise themselves with new situations.

9. Varied scenarios :
- Trainers vary the scenarios to expose nurses to a range of emergency situations and prepare them to respond to different medical conditions.

Emergency scenario simulations offer operating room nurses a valuable opportunity to learn, practise and develop their crisis management skills. This practical approach improves nurses' preparedness to respond effectively to unforeseen medical situations, contributing to patient safety and quality of care in the operating theatre.

Patient safety management

Checking patient identification protocols prior to surgery is a crucial step in ensuring the safety and integrity of the surgical process. Operating theatre nurses play an essential role in this check, ensuring that the right patient is undergoing the right surgical procedure and that all the necessary information is correct. Here's how they do it:

1. Preoperative check :
- Before surgery begins, the nurses confirm the patient's identity by comparing the information on his or her identification bracelet with the data in the medical record.

2. Confirmation by the patient :
- Nurses ask patients to confirm their name, date of birth and other crucial identifying information.

3. Checking the planned operation :
- The nurses ensure that the planned surgical procedure is consistent with the patient's information and that there is no confusion.

4. Comparison with documents :
- Nurses check documents such as informed consents, medical prescriptions and diagnostic reports to confirm the accuracy of the information.

5. Communication with the team :
   - Nurses communicate with the surgical team, including surgeons, anaesthetists and operating assistants, to ensure that everyone is aware of the patient's identity and procedure.

6. Using barcodes :
   - In many hospitals, barcodes are used to scan patient identification wristbands, medicines and surgical instruments, helping to prevent errors.

7. Double-checking :
   - In some cases, a double check is carried out by two members of the team to improve accuracy.

8. Error correction :
   - If inconsistencies or errors are identified, the nurses take steps to correct the situation before the surgery begins.

9. Documentation :
   - All the verification steps and results are carefully documented in the patient's medical file.

10. Safety awareness :
   - Nurses educate patients about the verification process and the importance of guaranteeing their identity and safety.

Checking patient identification protocols before surgery is standard practice to avoid medical errors and ensure patient safety. Operating room nurses are responsible for this thorough check, and in so doing they help to ensure the success of every surgical procedure.

Preventing medication errors and incorrect procedures in the operating theatre is an absolute priority for nurses. Medication errors and incorrect procedures can have serious consequences for patients and compromise their safety. Operating theatre nurses take a number of steps to minimise the risks and ensure that medication is administered safely and procedures are carried out accurately. Here's how they prevent these errors:

1. Checking medicines :
   - Nurses check medicines carefully before administration, comparing the label with the prescription and confirming the patient's identity.

2. Clear labelling :
   - Medicines are clearly and accurately labelled, including the name of the medicine, the dose, the method of administration and the time.

3. Double check :
   - In certain critical situations, the medication is double-checked by two members of the team to ensure accuracy.

4. Using barcodes :
   - Barcodes are often used to scan medicines and patient identification wristbands, reducing the risk of error.

5. Documentation :
   - Each administration of medication is accurately documented in the patient's medical file.

6. Allergy sensitisation :
   - Nurses find out about the patient's allergies before administering any medication and take steps to avoid drugs to which the patient is allergic.

7. Compliance with protocols :
   - Nurses rigorously follow established protocols for administering medicines, paying particular attention to doses, frequency and routes of administration.

8. Continuing education :
   - Nurses keep abreast of new information on medicines and take part in ongoing training to maintain their skills.

9. Standardised procedures :
   - Surgical and medicinal procedures are standardised and based on recognised guidelines to minimise variations and errors.

10. Interdisciplinary communication :
   - Nurses communicate effectively with members of the surgical team to ensure that everyone is aware of the

drugs being administered and the procedures being carried out.

11. Reporting errors :
  • If an error occurs, the nurses immediately report it to the medical team and the risk management department so that corrective action can be taken.

Preventing medication errors and incorrect procedures is a responsibility shared by the entire surgical team. Nurses play a central role in implementing rigorous measures to ensure patient safety in the operating theatre.

Staff safety management

Protocols for the safe handling of sharp instruments and equipment in the operating theatre are essential to prevent injuries and infections for both nurses and the surgical team. Sharp instruments and equipment used in surgery can represent a potential risk if they are not handled correctly. Here's how operating theatre nurses follow protocols to ensure safe handling:

1. Appropriate use of instruments :
  • Nurses are trained to use each instrument correctly, knowing its functions, specific use and precautions for use.

2. Preoperative preparation :
  • Sharp instruments and equipment are checked before surgery to ensure that they are sterile, in good condition and ready to use.

3. Handle with care :
  • Nurses handle sharp instruments using appropriate gripping techniques to minimise the risk of cuts.

4. Trays and work areas :
  • Instruments are arranged in an organised manner on sterile trays, and nurses take care not to move them unnecessarily to avoid contamination.

5. Use of pliers :
   - Nurses use forceps to grip sharp instruments and pass them to members of the surgical team, reducing the risk of injury.

6. Handling sutures :
   - Sutures and threads are handled with care to avoid unnecessary exposure to sharp points.

7. Use of special boxes :
   - The sharp instruments used, such as needles, are placed in special boxes designed to protect them during surgery and ensure their safe disposal.

8. Instrument recount :
   - At the end of the surgery, the nurses recount the instruments to ensure that no instrument has been left inside the patient.

9. Safe disposal :
   - Sharp instruments and equipment are disposed of safely in accordance with biomedical waste management protocols.

10. Wearing appropriate gloves :
   - Nurses wear appropriate gloves when handling sharp instruments or potentially contaminated material.

11. Sterile environment awareness :
   - Nurses are aware of the sterile environment around them and take precautions to avoid any non-sterile contact with instruments and equipment.

12. Continuing education and training :
   - Nurses receive ongoing training on best practice in the safe handling of instruments and equipment.

Safe handling of sharp instruments and equipment in the operating theatre is fundamental to preventing injury and the risk of infection. Strict protocols and proper practices ensure that the surgical process is carried out safely for patients and the medical team.

Preventing injuries and exposure to body fluids is a major priority in the operating theatre to ensure the safety of nurses and the medical team. Injuries from sharp objects, splashes of body fluids and accidental contact with biological materials present health and safety risks. Here's how operating theatre nurses prevent these injuries and exposures:

1. Use of personal protective equipment (PPE) :
   • Nurses wear gloves, masks, goggles and sterile coats to minimise contact with body fluids and contaminants.

2. Careful handling of instruments :
   • Sharp instruments are handled with care, using appropriate gripping techniques to avoid cuts.

3. Techniques for the safe removal of gloves :
   • Nurses are trained in safe glove removal techniques to avoid contamination when removing gloves.

4. Use of special containers :
   • Sharp instruments and objects are placed in special containers designed to prevent injury during disposal.

5. Handling precautions :
   • Nurses avoid handling sharp objects or piercing materials unnecessarily, thereby minimising the risk of injury.

6. Environmental awareness :
   • Nurses are aware of their surroundings and the proximity of potentially dangerous sharp objects or medical devices.

7. Use of barriers :
   • Protective barriers, such as sterile drapes and screens, are used to prevent splashes of body fluids.

8. Handling body fluids :
   • Nurses handle body fluids with care, avoiding splashes or direct contact.

9. Use of safety syringes :
   • Safety syringes with locking mechanisms are used to minimise the risk of accidental pricks.

- 10. Cardiopulmonary resuscitation (CPR) training:Nurses are trained in CPR to intervene rapidly in the event of serious injury.

11. Continuing education :
  - Nurses receive ongoing training on best practice in injury and exposure prevention.

12. Reporting incidents :
  - Any incident of injury or exposure is reported immediately so that appropriate action can be taken.

Preventing injury and exposure to body fluids is an essential aspect of operating theatre safety. Strict protocols and proper practices help to minimise risks to nurses and maintain a safe environment for all members of the medical team.

Quality control and performance assessment

Implementing measures to ensure compliance with operating theatre safety standards is essential to guarantee the safety of patients, the medical team and nurses. These measures aim to maintain a safe environment and prevent potential risks. Here's how OR nurses implement these measures:

1. Training and education :
  - Nurses receive initial and ongoing training on safety protocols, best practice and current standards.

2. Adherence to protocols :
  - The nurses rigorously follow the protocols established for each stage of the surgery, paying particular attention to safety procedures.

3. Use of personal protective equipment (PPE) :
  - Nurses wear the appropriate PPE, including gloves, masks, goggles and sterile coats, in accordance with standards.

4. Preoperative check :
  - Before surgery begins, the nurses carry out thorough checks to ensure that all protocols and safety measures are in place.

5. Interdisciplinary communication :
  - Nurses work closely with other members of the surgical team to ensure that everyone is aware of safety protocols.

6. Compliance with sterile procedures :
  - Nurses follow strict procedures to maintain a sterile environment, including wearing appropriate clothing and keeping instruments sterile.

7. Cross-contamination control :
  - Nurses take steps to avoid cross-contamination by using sterile drapes, barriers and disinfection protocols.

8. Biomedical waste management :
  - Nurses dispose of biomedical waste in accordance with waste management protocols to prevent the risk of contamination.

9. Monitoring vital signs :
  - Nurses constantly monitor the patient's vital signs during surgery to detect any changes quickly.

10. Patient identification :
- The nurses carefully check the patient's identification before surgery to ensure that the procedure is correct.

11. Infection prevention :
  - Nurses follow rigorous sterilisation, asepsis and infection prevention protocols to minimise risks.

12. Incident reports :
  - Safety incidents or potential errors are reported and documented for analysis and continuous improvement.

Implementing these measures ensures compliance with operating theatre safety standards, reducing the risks to patients and the medical team. This helps to maintain a safe and effective environment for surgical procedures.

Collecting data and analysing incidents in the operating theatre are essential practices to ensure continuous improvement in safety, quality of care and procedures. The data collected and analyses carried out enable problem areas to be identified, corrective measures to be put in place and future incidents to be prevented. Here's how operating theatre nurses carry out this process:

1. Data collection :
   • Nurses collect data on surgical incidents, errors, practices, procedures and outcomes.

2. Incident reporting :
   • Safety incidents, medical errors and adverse events are reported and documented in detailed reports.

3. Retrospective analysis :
   • Nurses analyse incidents using methods such as root cause analysis to identify contributing factors.

4. Risk Management Committee :
   • The data is reviewed by a Risk Management Committee, which assesses incidents, recommends corrective measures and monitors their implementation.

5. Case studies :
   • Incidents are examined in the form of case studies to understand the circumstances, human factors and processes involved.

6. Identifying trends :
   • The data is analysed to identify recurring trends, patterns and areas of risk.

7. Implementation of corrective measures :
   • Based on the analyses, corrective measures are put in place to prevent similar incidents from recurring.

8. Training and awareness :
   • The findings of the analyses are used to develop training and awareness programmes to improve the skills and safety awareness of the team.

9. Evaluation of protocols :
- Safety protocols and procedures are evaluated on the basis of the results of incident analyses to ensure their effectiveness.

10. Feedback :
- Nurses share their experiences and learning from incidents to promote a culture of learning and continuous improvement.

11. Monitoring performance indicators :
- Performance indicators are monitored and evaluated to measure progress and the effectiveness of corrective measures implemented.
12. Interdisciplinary communication :
- The conclusions of the analyses are communicated to the entire surgical team to ensure a collective understanding of the lessons learned.

By collecting data and analysing incidents, we can identify potential problems, take proactive measures and constantly improve operating theatre processes and protocols. This helps to create a safer environment for patients and medical staff.

Communication and coordination in the event of complications

Rapid and effective communication in the event of complications or incidents in the operating theatre is crucial to ensure a rapid response, minimise risks to patients and ensure coordination of the medical team. Nurses play a central role in this communication to ensure that problems are reported and managed quickly. Here's how they ensure fast and effective communication:

1. Use of dedicated communication systems :
- Operating theatres are often equipped with specific communication systems, such as intercoms or wireless communication devices, to enable instant communication between team members.

2. Communication hierarchy :
   - Nurses follow a defined communication hierarchy to report problems to the appropriate members of the medical team, usually starting with the anaesthetist or surgeon.

3. Verbal communication :
   - Nurses use verbal communication to report complications or incidents quickly, providing clear and precise information about the situation.

4. Using emergency codes :
   - Specific emergency codes are used to quickly signal critical situations, such as cardiac arrest or haemorrhage, and mobilise the entire medical team.

5. Use of manual signs :
   - Nurses can use pre-agreed hand signals to discreetly signal problems or needs to other team members.

6. Written communication :
   - Nurses immediately document any complications or incidents in the patient's medical file to ensure follow-up and continuity of care.

7. Regular team meetings :
   - The medical teams hold regular meetings to discuss cases, complications and incidents, which facilitates communication and collective learning.

8. Transfer of brief information :
   - Nurses communicate succinctly but thoroughly, so that essential information can be passed on quickly without delaying necessary action.

9. Constructive feedback :
   - After a complication has been resolved, the nurses take part in debriefings to discuss the actions taken, the results and the lessons learned.

10. Use of technology :
   - Electronic medical record management systems and secure communication applications can be used to share critical information rapidly.

11. Communication training :
  • Nurses receive training in interpersonal communication and conflict management to improve their ability to communicate effectively in stressful situations.

Rapid and effective communication in the event of complications or incidents enables the medical team to react quickly, make informed decisions and provide the best possible care for the patient. This helps to maintain the safety and quality of care in the operating theatre.

Coordinating efforts to resolve problems and stabilise the situation in the operating theatre is essential to ensure patient safety and a smooth surgical procedure. Nurses play a central role in this coordination, working closely with members of the medical team. Here's how they coordinate efforts to resolve problems and stabilise the situation:

1. Clear and concise communication :
  • Nurses communicate clearly and concisely with team members to share relevant information about the situation and the action to be taken.

2. Role of coordination nurses :
  • Some nurses may be designated as coordinating nurses, responsible for centralising information, organising resources and facilitating communication.

3. Definition of roles and responsibilities :
  • Each member of the team knows his or her role and responsibilities in the event of a problem, which facilitates a coordinated response.

4. Collective decision-making :
  • Major decisions are taken collectively, involving all team members to ensure a holistic approach.

5. Use of emergency protocols :
  • Pre-established emergency protocols are activated to guide actions in the event of major complications, ensuring a coherent and structured response.

6. Rapid mobilisation of resources :
   - The nurses coordinate the rapid mobilisation of the necessary resources, such as the anaesthesia team, advisory specialists, etc.

7. Prioritisation of actions :
   - The actions to be taken are prioritised according to urgency and impact on the patient, ensuring that the most critical measures are taken first.

8. Time management :
   - The nurses monitor the time carefully to ensure that the necessary actions are taken without undue delay.

9. Interdisciplinary collaboration :
   - Team members work closely together, sharing their expertise and knowledge to solve problems holistically.

10. Ongoing communication :
   - Nurses maintain ongoing communication with team members to keep everyone informed of developments and actions in progress.

11. Evaluation of effectiveness :
   - The nurses monitor the effectiveness of the measures taken and make any necessary adjustments as the situation evolves.

12. Debriefing after the resolution :
   - Once the problem has been resolved, the medical team meets for a debriefing to analyse the actions taken, identify lessons learned and explore opportunities for improvement.

Effective coordination of efforts to resolve problems and stabilise the situation is essential to minimise risks, ensure patient safety and guarantee the success of the operation. Nurses play a central role in this coordination, working with the entire medical team.

Integrating technologies for safety

The use of real-time patient monitoring and surveillance systems in the operating theatre is an essential practice for closely monitoring the patient's condition throughout the surgical procedure. These systems provide vital information in real time, enabling nurses and the medical team to detect changes quickly and take appropriate action. Here's how nurses use these systems:

1. Vital signs monitors :
    - The monitors monitor the patient's vital signs in real time, such as heart rate, blood pressure, oxygen saturation, temperature and respiratory rate.

2. Central screens :
    - The central screens display the vital signs of several patients simultaneously, enabling nurses to monitor several patients at the same time.

3. Alarms :
    - Monitoring systems issue alarms in the event of abnormal values or significant fluctuations in vital signs, alerting nurses to any problems.

4. Trend curves :
    - Trend curves are plotted in real time, enabling nurses to visualise changes in vital signs over a given period.

5. Customisable parameters :
    - Nurses can customise the alarm parameters to suit the specific needs of the patient and the surgical procedure.

6. Monitoring anaesthesia :
    - The monitoring systems also track anaesthetic-related parameters, such as the concentration of anaesthetic agents and the depth of anaesthesia.

7. Neurological monitoring :
    - For some surgeries, real-time neurological monitoring, such as electroencephalography (EEG), can be used to detect brain changes.

8. Haemodynamic monitoring :
   - Haemodynamic monitoring devices such as the pulmonary arterial line can be used to monitor the patient's haemodynamic parameters.

9. Blood gas monitoring :
   - Nurses monitor blood gas levels, including arterial blood gases and electrolytes, to assess acid-base balance.

10. Digital recordings :
   - The data is recorded digitally, enabling nurses to view and compare vital sign data over time.

11. Integration with medical records :
   - Monitoring systems can be integrated with electronic medical records for complete and accurate documentation.

12. Quick answer :
   - By monitoring data in real time, nurses can react quickly to sudden changes or complications.

The use of real-time patient monitoring and surveillance systems enables nurses to remain constantly informed of the patient's condition during surgery. This helps to guarantee patient safety and to take immediate action if necessary, ensuring optimum care in the operating theatre.

The adoption of advanced technologies in the operating theatre plays a crucial role in reducing human error and improving overall patient safety. These technologies are designed to complement the skills of healthcare professionals, minimise risk and optimise processes. Here's how nurses can adopt these technologies to reduce human error in the operating theatre:

1. Automated tracking systems :
   - Automated systems for monitoring vital signs and physiological data can rapidly detect abnormal variations and trigger alarms in the event of a problem.

2. Decision support systems :
   - Decision support software provides recommendations based on patient data, helping nurses to make informed decisions.

3. Surgical robotics :
   - Surgical robots assist surgeons and nurses in complex procedures, improving precision and reducing errors.

4. Advanced medical imaging :
   - Real-time imaging, such as intra-operative radiography and ultrasound, helps nurses to visualise the patient's internal structures during surgery.

5. Electronic medical records (EMR) :
   - EMRs provide instant access to patient information, reducing the errors associated with manual transcription.

6. Automated tagging and identification :
   - Automated patient identification and sample labelling systems reduce the risk of mistaken identity.

7. Intelligent instrumentation :
   - Intelligent surgical instruments can track the use and location of instruments, minimising the risk of objects being left inside the patient.

8. Augmented reality and virtual reality :
   - These technologies help nurses to visualise anatomical structures in 3D, facilitating navigation during complex procedures.

9. Simulation and virtual training :
   - Virtual simulators allow nurses to train for complex scenarios, improving their skills and decision-making.

10. Traceability of medicines and equipment :
   - Traceability systems guarantee the correct use of medicines and equipment, minimising the risk of errors.

11. Remote monitoring :
   - Telemedicine technologies allow nurses to monitor patients remotely, which can be useful in certain contexts.

12. Data analysis and machine learning :
   - Data analysis and machine learning can help identify trends, predict complications and improve decision-making.

Integrating these advanced technologies into the practice of operating theatre nurses can significantly reduce human error, improve patient safety and enhance the efficiency of care. However, it is important to note that these technologies must be used in a way that complements human skills and takes account of the clinical expertise of healthcare professionals.

Training and development of safety skills

Continuing education is essential for operating theatre nurses to improve their risk management and safety skills. Constant advances in the medical field, surgical techniques and safety standards require continuous updating of knowledge and skills. Here's how continuing education can help improve risk management and safety in the operating theatre:

1. Updating knowledge :
   • Ongoing training enables nurses to keep abreast of the latest medical advances, safety protocols and best practice.

2. Training in new technologies :
   • Nurses are trained in the safe use of new medical technologies and advanced equipment in the operating theatre.

3. Prevention techniques :
   • The training programmes cover specific techniques for preventing errors, complications and risks in the operating theatre.

4. Training in emergency procedures :
   • Nurses are trained in emergency management and rapid decision-making to ensure patient safety.

5. Practical simulations :
   • Complex scenario simulations help nurses to develop their risk management skills in a controlled environment.

6. Analysis of incidents :
   • Training can include analysis of past incidents to identify causes and preventive measures.

7. Effective communication :
   - Nurses are trained to communicate effectively in crisis situations, with an emphasis on coordination and collaboration.

8. Resource management :
   - Ongoing training may include modules on the effective management of material and human resources in the operating theatre.

9. Knowledge of protocols :
   - Nurses are trained in specific safety protocols, such as patient identification, pre-operative checks, etc.

10. Safety culture :
- Ongoing training encourages the creation of a culture of safety in the operating theatre, where every member of the team prioritises patient safety.

11. Stress management training :
- Nurses can be trained to manage stress and emotions during critical situations to maintain mental clarity.

12. Participation in workshops and conferences :
- Workshops and conferences offer the opportunity to learn from industry experts and exchange experiences with other professionals.

Continuing education plays a vital role in the professional development of operating theatre nurses, improving their risk management skills, enhancing their understanding of safety protocols and helping them to deliver high quality patient care.

Participation in workshops and best practice training is an important component of continuing education for operating theatre nurses. These learning opportunities provide an effective means of acquiring new skills, updating existing knowledge and learning about the latest approaches to safety and quality of care. Here's how participation in such workshops and training can benefit operating theatre nurses:

1. Acquiring new skills :
   - Workshops and training courses expose nurses to new techniques, technologies and approaches that can be implemented to improve the safety and quality of care.

2. Updating knowledge :
   - Nurses are kept abreast of the latest medical advances, updated clinical guidelines and new regulations relating to the operating theatre.

3. Sharing experiences :
   - The workshops provide an opportunity to share experiences and challenges with other nurses, encouraging mutual learning.

4. Interaction with experts :
   - Training courses are often led by industry experts, offering a unique opportunity to interact with seasoned professionals.

5. Practical application :
   - Workshops and training courses generally focus on real-life scenarios, enabling nurses to practise their newly acquired skills.

6. Strengthening decision-making :
   - Nurses learn to make informed decisions based on best practice and current scientific evidence.

7. Safety awareness :
   - Best practice training often emphasises the importance of patient safety, helping nurses to maintain a culture of safety.

8. Adapting to change :
   - The workshops help nurses to adapt quickly to changes in medical practice and integrate new approaches into their routine.

9. Professional networking :
   - Training events provide a platform for networking with other healthcare professionals and encourage knowledge sharing.

10. Implementation of improved protocols :
  • Nurses can learn to implement improved protocols and procedures to optimise care in the operating theatre.

11. Validation of skills :
  • Taking part in workshops can help validate skills and compliance with safety standards.

Attending workshops and training courses on best practice is a valuable investment for operating theatre nurses, as it prepares them to provide high-quality care, maintain patient safety and stay at the forefront of medical developments.

Chapter 5:
Communication and coordination in the operating theatre

The importance of effective communication in the operating theatre

Effective communication plays a crucial role in patient safety and surgical outcomes in the operating theatre. Clear, open and coordinated communication between all members of the medical team helps to minimise errors, prevent complications and ensure high quality care. Here's how communication impacts patient safety and surgical outcomes:

1. Error prevention :
   • Accurate communication helps to share vital information, avoid misunderstandings and prevent errors relating to medication, patient identification and so on.

2. Team coordination :
   • Effective communication facilitates the coordination of actions between surgeons, anaesthetists, nurses and other team members, ensuring that the surgical procedure runs smoothly.

3. Rapid response to complications :
   • Rapid communication in the event of complications means that decisions can be taken quickly and in a coordinated fashion to minimise the risks to the patient.

4. Emergency management :
   • Communication is essential to coordinate actions in emergency situations, such as cardiac arrest or excessive bleeding.

5. Transmission of preoperative information :
   • Accurate communication of pre-operative medical information, such as allergies, medication taken and

previous health problems, is essential in order to adapt care.

6. Monitoring vital signs :
   • Regular communication of the patient's vital signs between members of the team helps to monitor the patient's condition and detect any changes quickly.

7. Informed consent :
   • Clear and comprehensible communication between the medical team and the patient is essential to obtain informed consent for surgery.

8. Exchange of information :
   • Ongoing communication between team members ensures that important information is passed on throughout the procedure.

9. Preoperative preparation :
   - Communication between the medical team to prepare the patient, check the instruments and plan the surgery ensures efficient execution.

10. Post-operative follow-up :
    • Post-operative communication between the medical team is important for managing post-operative care and preventing complications.

11. Interdisciplinary collaboration :
    • Communication facilitates collaboration between different medical specialities, improving overall patient care.

12. Report and debriefing :
    • Communication at the end of surgery, during the report and debriefing, enables essential information to be shared for post-operative care.

Effective communication in the operating theatre helps to create a culture of safety, fosters trust within the medical team and improves surgical outcomes by ensuring consistent, well-coordinated, patient-centred care.

Communication in the surgical environment can be particularly complex due to a number of specific challenges. These challenges can have an impact on patient safety, team coordination and surgical outcomes. The following is an assessment of the key challenges related to communication in the surgical environment:

1. Professional hierarchy :
   - The medical hierarchy can sometimes inhibit open communication, especially if team members are reluctant to express their concerns or suggestions to more experienced professionals.

2. Stress and time pressure :
   - The stressful environment of the operating theatre can make it difficult to communicate clearly and thoughtfully, leading to misunderstandings and mistakes.

3. Non-verbal communication :
   - Because of masks, goggles and other equipment, non-verbal communication, such as facial expressions, can be limited, making it more difficult to understand emotions and intentions.

4. Multi-tasking :
   - Team members often have to juggle many simultaneous tasks, which can make coherent and timely communication difficult.

5. Environmental noise :
   - Noise from equipment, conversations and alarms in the operating theatre can disrupt communication and prevent attentive listening.

6. Staff changes :
   - The frequent rotation of medical and nursing staff can lead to problems of familiarity and mutual understanding.

7. Language and cultural barriers :
   - Surgical teams can be made up of members from different cultures and languages, which can lead to communication difficulties.
8. Incomplete information transfer :
   - Important information may be omitted or poorly transmitted when moving from one member of the team to

116

another (such as the change from the surgical team to the post-operative care team).

9. Use of abbreviations and jargon :
   • Excessive use of abbreviations and medical jargon can lead to misunderstandings, particularly for team members less familiar with these terms.

10. Asynchronous communication :
    • Team members may not always be present in the operating theatre at the same time, which can lead to problems with the transmission of information.

11. Emergency communication :
    • Emergency situations require rapid, coordinated communication, which can be difficult to achieve under pressure.

12. Complex information transfer :
    • Communicating complex medical information, such as the details of a procedure, may require specific communication skills to ensure understanding.

To overcome these challenges, it is crucial to implement effective communication strategies, such as pre-operative briefings, audit protocols, training in inter-professional communication and raising awareness of the importance of open and respectful communication within the surgical team.

Roles and responsibilities within the surgical team

Clarity of roles within the surgical team, comprising surgeons, anaesthetists, nurses and operating assistants, is essential to ensure effective coordination, minimise errors and guarantee patient safety. Each member of the team has specific responsibilities that contribute to the success of the surgical procedure. Here is an overview of the roles of each group:

Surgeons:
    • Surgeons are responsible for carrying out the surgical procedure. Their medical and technical expertise is crucial

to carrying out the procedure safely and effectively. Surgeons' responsibilities include planning the procedure, performing the surgical procedures, making intraoperative decisions and communicating with the team.

Anaesthetists:
- Anaesthetists are responsible for managing the patient's anaesthesia during surgery. Their role is to assess the patient's state of health, choose the appropriate method of anaesthesia, administer the necessary drugs and continuously monitor the patient's vital signs during the procedure. They play a key role in maintaining the patient's physiological stability.

Operating theatre nurses :
- Operating theatre nurses have a diverse role that includes preparing the operating theatre, managing instruments and sterile equipment, assisting the surgeon and anaesthetist, monitoring the patient's vital signs, ensuring accurate documentation and coordinating the team. They ensure that all logistical and clinical aspects of the procedure run smoothly.

Operating aids :
- Operating assistants, often referred to as surgical technicians, provide direct practical support to surgeons. Their duties include handling instruments, maintaining a sterile field, taking specimens and carrying out specific tasks according to the surgeon's needs. They ensure a safe and efficient workflow during the procedure.

To ensure clarity of roles and smooth communication, it is important that each member of the team understands not only their own role, but also those of others. Pre-operative briefings, audit protocols, inter-professional communication training and regular meetings can help to reinforce mutual understanding of roles and create a collaborative and safe working environment. When every member of the team is clear about what is expected of them, the quality of care and patient outcomes improve significantly.

Interprofessional collaboration is a crucial component of holistic patient management in the surgical environment. It involves close cooperation and effective communication between the various members of the medical team, including surgeons, anaesthetists, nurses, operating theatre assistants and other health professionals. This comprehensive approach ensures that all aspects of the patient's health and well-being are taken into account, from preparation for surgery through to post-operative recovery. Here's how interprofessional collaboration ensures holistic patient care:

1. Full assessment :
   - The team members bring their unique skills to bear on a comprehensive assessment of the patient, taking into account their medical condition, history, allergies, medication and any other relevant factors.

2. Preoperative planning :
   - Interprofessional collaboration enables the surgical procedure to be discussed and planned, taking into account all the medical, anaesthetic and logistical aspects to ensure patient safety and comfort.

3. Communicating the patient's needs :
   - The different professionals share essential information about the patient's specific needs, such as dietary preferences, medical restrictions and mobility problems.

4. Intra-operative coordination :
   - During surgery, inter-professional collaboration ensures real-time communication to respond to changing patient needs, adapt care and minimise risks.

5. Pain and anxiety management :
   - Professionals work together to manage the patient's pain and anxiety before, during and after the procedure, using both medicinal and non-medicinal approaches.

6. Post-operative monitoring and follow-up :
   - After surgery, collaboration continues to monitor the patient's recovery, administer the necessary medication, monitor vital signs and manage any complications.

7. Rehabilitation and recovery :
   - Team members work together to develop personalised rehabilitation plans and provide ongoing care to facilitate optimal patient recovery.

8. Communication with the patient and family :
   - Effective inter-professional communication ensures that patients and their families are well informed about the procedure, post-operative care and expectations, thereby fostering trust and understanding.

9. Transfer of care :
   - When the patient is ready to leave hospital, interprofessional collaboration ensures a smooth transition to post-operative care at home or in a rehabilitation facility.

Interprofessional collaboration enriches patient care by providing multidisciplinary expertise, avoiding information silos and ensuring a holistic, patient-centred approach. This improves the quality of care, reduces the risk of errors and contributes to optimal surgical and recovery outcomes.

Pre-operative briefing protocols

Preoperative meetings are an important step in the planning and coordination of surgical procedures. They bring together key members of the medical team, including surgeons, anaesthetists, operating theatre nurses, surgical assistants and other healthcare professionals involved in the procedure. The purpose of these meetings is to discuss the surgical plan, address concerns and ensure a common understanding of the upcoming procedure. Here's how preoperative meetings benefit surgical planning:

1. Review of the surgical plan :
   - Pre-operative meetings allow team members to review the details of the surgical plan, including the specific stages of the procedure, the planned incisions, patient positions, instruments required, etc.

2. Clarification of roles :
   - Each professional in the team understands their role in the procedure and how they will contribute to the success of the operation.

3. Discussion of concerns :
   - Team members have the opportunity to raise and discuss potential concerns, such as patient allergies, significant medical history, time constraints or other logistical issues.

4. Management of anticipated complications :
   - Pre-operative meetings are used to discuss potential complications and action plans in the event of an emergency.

5. Logistics coordination :
   - Logistical details such as the arrangement of instruments, the layout of the operating theatre and the specific needs of the patient are discussed to ensure that the procedure runs smoothly.

6. Interprofessional communication :
   - Preoperative meetings encourage interprofessional communication by enabling the different members to share their perspectives and specific knowledge.

7. Planning anaesthesia :
   - Anaesthetists can discuss the anaesthetic methods to be used, the drugs to be administered and the management of the patient's physiological stability during the procedure.

8. Collaborative decision-making :
   - Pre-operative meetings facilitate collaborative decision-making by identifying the best approaches for the procedure and taking into account the opinions of all team members.

9. Error reduction :
   - By anticipating challenges and clarifying details, pre-operative meetings help to reduce errors and misunderstandings during the procedure.

10. Building trust :
   • Pre-operative meetings foster trust and cohesion within the team by ensuring that all members understand the common objectives and are aligned on the surgical plan.

In short, preoperative meetings are a valuable tool for optimising planning, coordination and communication within the medical team, contributing to safer, more efficient and better coordinated surgery.

The exchange of crucial information is an essential element in establishing a common understanding of the objectives of the surgery within the medical team. Clear and precise communication allows each member of the team to understand the specific details of the surgical procedure, expectations and objectives to ensure a smooth and successful execution. Here's how the exchange of crucial information facilitates a common understanding of the objectives of the surgery:

1. Presentation of the case :
   • The exchange of information begins with a detailed presentation of the patient's case, including medical history, symptoms, test results and reasons for surgery.

2. Surgical plan :
   • Details of the surgical plan are shared, including the specific stages of the procedure, the incisions planned, the techniques to be used and the aims of the surgery.

3. Roles and responsibilities :
   • Each member of the team understands their role in the procedure and how they will contribute to achieving the objectives of the surgery.

4. Potential complications :
   • Information on potential complications and action plans in the event of an emergency is shared to ensure adequate preparation.

5. Anaesthesia and monitoring :
   • Anaesthetists share information on managing patient anaesthesia, monitoring vital signs and physiological stabilisation.

6. Pain management :
   - Intraoperative and postoperative pain management plans are communicated to ensure patient comfort and well-being.

7. Instruments and equipment :
   - Details of the specific instruments, medical devices and equipment required are shared to guarantee their availability and operation.

8. Patient details :
   - Crucial patient information, such as allergies, current medication and personal preferences, is exchanged to personalise care.

9. Transfer of care :
   - If necessary, plans for transferring post-operative care to the follow-up team are discussed to ensure optimum continuity of care.

10. Questions and concerns :
   - Team members have the opportunity to ask questions, express concerns and discuss important points to ensure full understanding.

The exchange of crucial information promotes a common understanding of the objectives of the surgery, strengthens team cohesion and reduces the risk of errors or misunderstandings during the procedure. It also creates an environment where every healthcare professional can contribute in an informed and proactive way to achieving the best outcomes for the patient.

Communication during surgery

Verbal and non-verbal communication techniques play an essential role in the operating theatre to ensure smooth coordination, mutual understanding and quality care. Given the complex and sometimes stressful environment of the operating theatre, effective communication is crucial to ensuring patient safety and the success of the surgical procedure. The following are examples of verbal and non-verbal communication techniques used in the operating theatre:

Verbal communication :

1. Pre-operative briefing: Before surgery begins, a briefing meeting can be organised to discuss the surgical plan, the roles of each team member and any concerns.

2. Announcement of stages: Surgeons and operating assistants announce the stages of the procedure as they progress to keep all team members informed.

3. Confirmation of actions : The team can use confirmation phrases such as "I confirm" or "I'm ready" to indicate that the planned steps have been completed.

4. Exchange of critical information: Professionals share crucial information, such as test results, changes in the patient's condition or adjustments to the procedure.

5. Ask for clarification: If an instruction is unclear, team members can ask for clarification using phrases such as "Can you repeat that?" or "Can you elaborate?"

6. Reporting anomalies: If something does not seem to be in line with the plan, team members should feel comfortable reporting anomalies using direct but respectful language.

7. Communication with the patient : Professionals can explain the forthcoming procedure to the patient, speak gently to reassure them and answer any questions they may have.

Non-verbal communication :

1. Eye contact: Establish and maintain eye contact with other team members to show attention and understanding.

2. Hand gestures: Use hand gestures to indicate specific actions or give instructions.

3. Facial expressions: Facial expressions can show approval, concern or other emotions, contributing to mutual understanding.

4. Body language: Open, team-oriented body language can convey an attitude of cooperation and listening.

5. Head movements: A nod of the head can signify approval, understanding or confirmation.

6. Use of spatial cues: The position and orientation of team members in the operating theatre can indicate intentions or needs.

7. Expressing calm: Maintaining a calm gait and posture can help create a serene environment despite stressful situations.

8. Use of silences: Intentional moments of silence can indicate the need to concentrate or pay attention to a specific task.

By combining verbal and non-verbal communication techniques, the surgical team can create a fluid and complete flow of information, which is essential for patient safety and the success of the procedure. Open, respectful and well-coordinated communication strengthens mutual trust and collaboration within the team.

Effective reporting of changes in the patient's condition and potential problems in the operating theatre is of paramount importance to ensure patient safety and well-being. Members of the medical team must be able to communicate quickly and clearly to report any abnormalities or concerns. Here are some steps and guidelines for effective reporting:

1. Use direct and concise communication: When reporting a change in the patient's condition or a potential problem, be direct and concise in your communication. Use clear, specific language to convey the information.

2. Identify yourself and your role: When you report a problem, start by identifying yourself and your role within the team. This helps establish the source of the information and facilitates coordination.

3. Use the communication protocol: Many hospitals and healthcare facilities have specific communication protocols for reporting changes in a patient's condition. Make sure you follow these protocols to ensure that the information is transmitted correctly.

4. Provide specific details: When reporting a problem, include specific details such as relevant vital signs, symptoms observed, location of the problem and any other relevant details.

5. Use visual tools if possible: If possible, use visual tools such as graphs, diagrams or images to illustrate the problem or changes. This can help clarify information and convey the situation quickly.

6. Be aware of the context: When reporting a problem, make sure you provide the necessary context for other team members to understand the bigger picture.

7. State the urgency: If the situation requires immediate attention, make sure you state this clearly. Use words like "urgent" or "immediate" to emphasise the seriousness of the situation.

8. Propose solutions if possible: If you have ideas or suggestions for solving the problem, don't hesitate to share them. Working together to find solutions is essential to ensure that the problem is dealt with quickly and effectively.

9. Listen carefully to feedback: When you report a problem, be prepared to listen to feedback from other team members. Communication is a two-way process, and it's important to remain open to comments and additional information.

10. Document the report : After reporting a change in the patient's condition or a potential problem, be sure to document the information appropriately in the patient's medical record. This will ensure that the situation is followed up accurately.

By following these guidelines, you can contribute to effective communication and rapid management of potential problems in the operating theatre, which is essential for patient safety and well-being.

Cooperation during care transitions

The transfer of information when teams and surgical phases change is a critical step in ensuring continuity of care and patient safety. When different teams or surgical phases change, it is essential that relevant information about the patient, the surgical plan, potential complications and other crucial details is passed on accurately and completely. Here's how to facilitate effective information transfer:

1. Pre-operative briefing: Before surgery begins, organise a pre-operative briefing where the outgoing team informs the incoming team of key details about the patient, the surgical plan and any special concerns.

2. Use structured communication: Use structured communication tools such as SBAR (Situation, Background, Assessment, Recommendation) to organise and convey information clearly and systematically.

3. Clearly identify the team members: When transferring information, make sure that each team member introduces himself and indicates his role to establish a clear identification.

4. Writing and reading reports: If possible, provide the incoming team with a written report containing essential information about the patient, changes during surgery, measures taken and any concerns.

5. Use visual aids: Diagrams, images and anatomical models can be useful to visually show key aspects of the procedure or areas of interest.

6. Include relevant information: Pass on important information such as the patient's vital signs, details of the surgical plan, allergies, potential complications, medication adjustments and other crucial items.

7. Ensure mutual understanding: Encourage members of the outgoing team to ask questions of the incoming team to ensure that information is clear and understood.

8. Define the objectives to be achieved: If there are specific objectives to be achieved during the next phase of surgery, make sure you communicate them clearly.

9. Provide recommendations: If decisions or actions need to be taken by the incoming team, include specific recommendations to guide their next step.

10. Recap and summarise: At the end of the handover, briefly recap the key points to ensure that nothing important has been omitted.

11. Encourage open communication: Create an environment where team members feel comfortable asking questions, clarifying points and sharing concerns.

12. Document the transfer: Make sure you document the transfer of information in the patient's medical file to ensure accurate monitoring and traceability.

Smooth, accurate information transfer between teams and surgical phases is essential to maintain patient safety, avoid errors and ensure consistent, effective care.

Preventing errors during patient transfer from the operating theatre to the recovery room is a critical step in ensuring patient safety during the post-operative period. Patient transfer involves potential risks, particularly in terms of medical complications, changes in condition and communication. Here are some strategies for preventing errors during this crucial transfer:

1. Transparent communication : Ensure there is clear and accurate communication between the operating room team and the recovery room team. Use structured communication protocols such as SBAR to convey important patient information.

2. Transfer report: Provide a written or verbal transfer report detailing essential information, such as the patient's condition, surgical plan, medication administered, complications encountered, allergies, fluids administered, etc.

3. Use of checklists: Adopt transfer-specific checklists to ensure that all the required steps are followed correctly.

4. Verification of patient identity : Before transfer, confirm the patient's identity using at least two methods of identification, such as verification of identity bracelet, verification of name and date of birth, etc.

5. Continuous monitoring: Ensure that the patient is constantly monitored during the transfer to quickly detect any changes in condition or complications.

6. Preparation of the recovery room: Before the patient arrives, make sure that the recovery room is properly prepared with all the necessary equipment and medicines.

7. Communication of medication : Clearly communicate the medication administered during surgery to the recovery room team, specifying doses and times.

8. Continuity of anaesthesia: If the patient is under anaesthesia, ensure that there is fluid and transparent communication between the anaesthetist in the operating theatre and the recovery room team to ensure a smooth transition.

9. Communication about complications: If complications have arisen during surgery, ensure that the recovery room team is informed and prepared to manage these complications if they arise during the recovery period.

10. Training and awareness: Educate operating room and recovery room staff on transfer procedures and error prevention protocols. Provide ongoing training to update skills and knowledge.

11. Use of technological tools: Use technologies such as health information systems to document and share patient information securely and accurately.

12. Analysis of previous errors: Carry out regular case reviews to examine the errors or problems that occurred during previous transfers and identify areas for improvement.

Preventing errors during patient transfer from the operating theatre to the recovery room requires effective communication, close coordination between teams and meticulous attention to detail. By following clear protocols, fostering a culture of safety and implementing specific strategies, the risk of errors can be significantly reduced.

Conflict management and problem solving

Managing disagreement and conflict within the surgical team is essential to maintaining a harmonious working environment, ensuring patient safety and promoting effective decision-making. Disagreements and conflicts can arise due to a variety of factors, such as differing opinions on the surgical plan, concerns about the patient or interpersonal tensions. Here are some techniques for managing these situations constructively:

1. Open communication: Encourage open and respectful communication within the team. Allow each member to express themselves and explain their point of view in a calm and respectful manner.
2. Active listening: Listen carefully to the concerns and points of view of other team members. Show that you understand and take their opinions into account.

3. Find common ground: Try to find common ground by exploring areas of agreement and possible solutions. Look for mutually beneficial solutions.

4. Mediation: If the conflict persists, consider mediation. A neutral third party can help facilitate communication and find solutions.

5. Respect for roles and responsibilities: Make sure that everyone in the team understands and respects each other's roles and responsibilities. This can reduce conflicts arising from misunderstandings or overlaps.

6. Effective leadership: Strong leadership can play a crucial role in managing conflict. Leaders must be able to make informed decisions, listen to team members and resolve disagreements fairly.

7. Focus on the facts: When discussing a disagreement, base yourself on tangible facts rather than emotions. This can contribute to a more objective discussion.

8. Managing emotions : Learn to manage your emotions and those of others constructively. Avoid knee-jerk reactions and take time to think before you respond.

9. Choice of words: Use carefully chosen words to avoid aggravating the situation. Avoid offensive or accusatory comments.

10. Find patient-centred solutions: When there is a disagreement, always remember that the patient's well-being is the priority. This can help to put problems into perspective and find solutions.

11. Post-conflict evaluation: After the conflict has been resolved, take the time to evaluate what happened and the lessons you learned. This can help prevent similar conflicts in the future.

12. Conflict management training: Provide training for the team on conflict management and effective communication. This can build the team's skills and confidence in resolving disagreements.

By implementing these techniques and fostering a culture of open communication and mutual respect, disagreements and conflicts within the team can be managed constructively, contributing to a positive working environment and high-quality patient care.

Resolving problems quickly and maintaining a positive working environment within the surgical team is essential to ensure patient safety and team member satisfaction. Here are some approaches to achieving this effectively:

1. Open communication: Encourage open and transparent communication between team members. Create a space where everyone can express their concerns, ask questions and share ideas.

2. Anticipating problems: Identify potential problems before they occur. Proactive anticipation allows you to take preventive measures and avoid problems turning into critical situations.

3. Interdisciplinary collaboration: Involve members of the surgical team as well as other healthcare professionals, such as anaesthetists, nurses and operating theatre assistants, in problem-solving. An interdisciplinary approach can bring different perspectives and creative solutions.

4. Use of protocols and checklists: Put in place protocols and checklists to guide key steps in the surgical process. This can help minimise errors and ensure consistency of practice.

5. Ongoing training: Offer ongoing training to the team to keep their skills up to date and keep them abreast of new practices and technologies. A well-trained team is better equipped to solve problems.

6. Constructive feedback: Provide constructive feedback to team members, focusing on areas for improvement while acknowledging successes. This fosters a positive, learning environment.

7. Encourage reporting of incidents: Encourage team members to report incidents, errors or potential problems. An open reporting system means that problems can be dealt with quickly and corrective measures put in place.

8. Time management: Optimise time management to avoid delays and stressful situations. Effective planning can help prevent problems linked to time constraints.

9. Use of technology : Adopt digital technologies and tools to improve communication, documentation and information management. Computerised systems can make it easier to solve problems.

10. Solution-focused approach: When a problem arises, encourage the team to adopt a solution-focused approach rather than concentrating on the negative. Quickly identify what needs to be done to solve the problem.

11. Positive leadership: Leaders play a crucial role in maintaining a positive working environment. Leaders must model positive behaviour, foster collaboration and encourage proactive problem solving.

12. Celebrating success: Recognising and celebrating the team's successes strengthens motivation and cohesion. Successes help to maintain a positive and inspiring environment. By adopting these approaches, the surgical team can work together more effectively to resolve problems quickly, maintain a positive environment and ensure the safety and well-being of patients.

Communication with patients and families

Explaining surgical procedures and stages to patients and their families is an essential part of the operating theatre nurse's role. This communication provides patients and their families with clear information, answers their questions and reassures them about the surgical process. Here's how to do it effectively:

1. Preparation: Choose an appropriate, calm moment to explain the surgical procedure. Make sure the patient is relaxed and open to communication.

2. Use understandable language: Avoid complex medical jargon and use simple, understandable language. Explain medical terms if necessary.

3. Active listening: Before you start explaining, encourage the patient and those close to them to ask questions and express their concerns. Listen carefully to their needs and concerns.

4. Description of the procedure: Explain the surgical procedure in detail, including objectives, specific steps and instruments used. Use visual aids such as diagrams or anatomical models if this helps to clarify explanations.

5. Risks and benefits: Discuss the potential risks associated with the procedure, as well as the expected benefits. Explain possible alternatives if they exist.

6. Duration and recovery: Inform the patient about the approximate duration of the surgery and the stages of post-operative recovery. Mention the care needed and precautions to be taken after surgery.

7. Anaesthesia: Explain the type of anaesthetic that will be used and how the patient will feel during and after the procedure.

8. Lifestyle implications: If the procedure will have an impact on the patient's lifestyle, discuss this in detail. This may include activity restrictions, dietary changes, etc.

9. Answering questions: Encourage patients and their families to ask questions at any time. Answer honestly and completely.

10. Empathy and emotional support: Understand that the surgical procedure may arouse emotions in the patient and those close to them. Show empathy, offer emotional support and reassure them.

11. Provision of written material: If possible, provide brochures or written documents describing the procedure, the necessary preparations and post-operative information.

12. Confidentiality: Ensure that the information provided is confidential and respect the patient's privacy.

By providing clear explanations tailored to individual needs, you help patients and their families to better understand the surgical procedure, make informed decisions and feel supported throughout the process.

Providing emotional support and answering patients' questions are key to reducing anxiety before surgery. Anxiety can be very worrying for patients and can impact on their experience and recovery. Here's how you can provide effective emotional support and answer questions to help reduce anxiety:

1. Create a welcoming environment: Make sure the patient feels safe and comfortable. Create a calm, warm space where they can ask questions and express their concerns.

2. Establish a connection: Take the time to introduce yourself and establish a relationship of trust with the patient. Show empathy and understanding for their feelings.

3. Encourage questions: Let patients know that they can ask any questions they have. Reassure them that all their concerns will be addressed.

4. Active listening: When the patient is talking, listen carefully and show that you are really involved. This can help ease their worries.

5. Clarify information: If the patient expresses concerns based on incorrect or misunderstood information, explain and clarify the relevant points.

6. Use of visual aids: If possible, use visual aids such as brochures, explanatory videos or diagrams to illustrate the procedure and answer questions.

7. Explain the steps: Break the procedure down into steps and explain them to the patient. This can help demystify the process and reduce anxiety.

8. Answer honestly: Provide honest and precise answers to the patient's questions. If you don't know the answer, indicate that you will obtain the necessary information.

9. Expectation management: Help the patient understand what to expect before, during and after surgery. This can reduce surprises and uncertainties.

10. Relaxation techniques: Teach patients simple relaxation techniques, such as deep breathing or visualisation, to help them manage their anxiety.

11. Involve the family: If the patient wishes, involve the family or close friends in the information and emotional support process.

12. Follow-up: Make sure you remain available to the patient even after the initial discussion. Showing that you are there to answer any further questions can help relieve anxiety.

Emotional support and answers to questions not only help to reduce patient anxiety, but also establish a bond of trust between the patient and the medical team. This can contribute to a more positive patient experience and better surgical outcomes.

Use of communication technologies

The use of electronic communication systems and operating theatre dashboards can significantly improve the efficiency, coordination and safety of surgical procedures. These modern tools facilitate communication between members of the surgical team, allow real-time monitoring of vital information and contribute to the overall management of the operating theatre. Here's how these systems can benefit you and how they are used:

Electronic communication systems :
- **Instant messaging:** Team members can communicate quickly and discreetly via instant messaging systems on mobile devices. This allows important information to be transmitted without interrupting the workflow.

- **Video calls:** Real-time exchanges via video calls can enable surgeons to consult other experts remotely, obtain advice and share images live.

- **Emergency alerts:** Systems can be configured to send alerts in the event of emergency situations, such as changes in a patient's vital signs or technical problems.

- **Equipment management :** Communication systems can be used to monitor equipment status, report faults and request repairs quickly.

Operating theatre dashboards :
- **Real-time monitoring: Dashboards** display patient vital signs, anaesthetic levels, intravenous fluid information, etc. in real time, enabling the team to monitor the patient continuously.

136

- **Surgical planning: Dashboards** can display the surgical plan, radiological images and other relevant information so that the team can refer to this data during the operation.

- **Checklists:** Pre-operative and post-operative checklists can be integrated into the dashboards, helping to ensure that all steps are followed correctly.

- **Time management:** Dashboards can track surgery times, radiation exposure times, etc., helping to maintain punctuality.

- **Data integration:** Data from a variety of sources, such as medical equipment, electronic patient records and radiology images, can be integrated into the dashboard, providing a complete view of the situation.

- **Real-time documentation:** Important information can be entered directly into the dashboard, reducing the need for manual notes and making documentation easier.

The use of electronic communication systems and dashboards in the operating theatre can improve coordination, reduce errors, speed up responses to emergency situations and provide a database for post-operative analysis. However, it is important to ensure that these technologies are seamlessly integrated into existing workflows and that team members are properly trained in their use.

The integration of digital tools in the operating theatre can significantly improve communication and coordination within the surgical team. Modern technologies enable real-time information sharing, access to vital data and facilitate informed decision-making. Here's how digital tools can be integrated to improve communication and coordination in the operating theatre:

1. Electronic records management systems: Electronic patient records (EPRs) provide easy storage and access to patient medical information, including medical history, test results and prescriptions. Team members can consult this data to gain a better understanding of the patient's situation.

2. Interactive dashboards: Digital dashboards display key information in real time, such as vital signs, blood test results and radiology images. This allows the team to continuously monitor the patient's condition and make decisions quickly.

3. Messaging and communication systems: Secure messaging applications enable team members to communicate quickly and discreetly, whether via text, voice or video messages. This makes it easier to coordinate tasks and resolve problems.

4. Instrument tracking systems: RFID chips or barcodes can be used to track the location and use of surgical instruments, helping to prevent errors and ensure the availability of necessary equipment.

5. Augmented and virtual reality applications: These technologies can be used to display real-time information in the surgeon's field of vision, which can be particularly useful during complex procedures.

6. Surgical planning systems: Planning software allows surgeons to simulate and plan procedures prior to surgery, which can help anticipate challenges and make informed decisions.

7. Hands-free communication devices: Hands-free headphones and microphones allow team members to communicate while keeping their hands free, which is essential in the operating theatre.

8. Mobile applications: Mobile applications allow team members to stay connected and access important information even when they are on the move in the operating theatre.

9. Access to radiological images: Radiological images can be displayed on digital screens in the operating theatre, giving surgeons a clear, detailed view of anatomical structures.

10. Videoconferences: Videoconferences can be used to consult experts remotely and obtain advice in real time.

Integrating these digital tools can help streamline processes, reduce errors, improve communication and facilitate coordination between members of the surgical team. However, it is essential to ensure that these technologies are implemented correctly, that team members are trained in their use and that data confidentiality is respected.

Interprofessional communication training

Training programmes to develop effective communication skills in the operating theatre are essential to ensure smooth coordination, rapid decision-making and improved patient safety. Here is an overview of the key elements to be included in such programmes:

1. Verbal communication :
   - Active listening techniques to understand the needs and concerns of team members.
   - Practical for clearly articulating information and giving precise instructions.
   - Use of clear language tailored to the target audience, avoiding complex medical jargon.
   - Practising communication in stressful and urgent situations.
   -
2. Non-verbal communication :
   - The importance of facial expressions, body language and eye contact in reinforcing messages.

   - Understand how non-verbal signals can influence perception and understanding.

   - Managing vocal intonation and posture to convey professionalism and confidence.

3. Interpersonal communication :
   - Developing positive and respectful relationships within the surgical team.

   - Managing disagreements and conflicts constructively.

   - Working effectively with diverse personalities.

4. Team communication :
- Techniques for sharing information effectively with all team members.

- Use of structured communication methods, such as pre-operative briefing and post-operative debriefing.

- Practice in coordinating tasks and responsibilities between different roles.

5. Communication with patients and their families :
- Developing skills in clearly explaining surgical procedures to patients.

- Practising empathic communication and managing the emotions of patients and their families.

- Respond to questions and concerns with sensitivity and understanding.

6. Use of electronic communication tools :
- Training in the safe and effective use of messaging applications and electronic communication systems in the operating theatre.

7. Simulation of communication scenarios :
- Use of simulation scenarios to reproduce common and complex communication situations.
- Performance analysis and feedback to improve skills.

8. Cultural and linguistic awareness :
- Understanding the impact of culture and linguistic diversity on communication.

- Developing the skills needed to communicate effectively with patients from different cultural and linguistic backgrounds.

9. Stress management training :
- Techniques for maintaining clear communication and decision-making under pressure.
- Managing emotions and personal stress to maintain professional communication.

10. Continuous assessment :
  • Integration of ongoing training sessions to update and reinforce communication skills.

Integrating training in effective communication into the career path of operating theatre nurses can make a significant contribution to better coordination, increased patient safety and optimised surgical outcomes.

Real-time scenario simulation is a powerful tool for improving coordination and decision-making within the surgical team. It allows team members to practice and become familiar with the complex and unexpected situations that can arise during surgery. Here's how scenario simulation can be used to improve real-time coordination in the operating theatre:

1. Scenario selection: Identify critical or problematic situations that require close coordination. This could include medical emergencies, unexpected complications, changes to the surgical plan, etc.

2. Create a realistic environment: faithfully recreate the operating theatre environment using simulation mannequins, medical equipment and scenery. The more realistic the environment, the more beneficial the simulation experience.

3. Interdisciplinary simulation: Involve all members of the surgical team, including surgeons, anaesthetists, nurses and operating assistants. This reflects real working dynamics and improves interdisciplinary coordination.

4. Scenarios based on real cases: Design scenarios based on real cases that have posed coordination challenges in the past. This allows team members to practise specifically on problems they have encountered.

5. Integration of communication: Focus on communication between team members. Encourage the use of electronic communication systems, voice calls and non-verbal gestures to coordinate actions.

6. Emergency management: Incorporate emergency scenarios to help the team manage stressful situations and make rapid, appropriate decisions.

7. Supervision and debriefing: An experienced trainer can supervise the simulation, provide real-time advice and organise a debriefing after the simulation. Reflective analysis of actions taken and decisions made can help identify areas for improvement.

8. Variety of scenarios: Design a variety of scenarios to cover different aspects of coordination, role-specific challenges and levels of complexity.

9. Regular rehearsal: Organise simulation sessions on a regular basis to allow the team to practise and continually reinforce its coordination skills.

10. Use of technology: Some simulations can be carried out using virtual simulators or virtual reality, offering additional flexibility and training possibilities.

Real-time scenario simulation provides a safe environment for learning and practice, and enables the team to develop coordination, communication and decision-making skills. It also fosters cohesion and trust between team members, which is essential for a well-coordinated operating theatre.

Chapter 6:
Types of surgery and specific features

General surgery

General surgery is a surgical specialty that focuses on the surgical management of a variety of medical conditions. It covers a wide range of surgical areas, each with its own specific techniques, procedures and considerations. Here are some of the main areas of general surgery:

1. Abdominal surgery :
   - Appendectomy: Removal of the appendix.
   - Cholecystectomy: removal of the gallbladder.
   - Intestinal resection: removal of part of the intestine.
   - Herniorrhaphy: Repair of an inguinal, umbilical or ventral hernia.
   - Gastrectomy: partial or total removal of the stomach.

2. Thoracic surgery :
   - Pulmonary lobectomy: removal of a lobe of the lung.
   - Thoracic tumour resection: removal of tumours from the thoracic cavity.
   - Chest wall surgery: Correction of deformities or injuries to the chest wall.

3. Vascular surgery :
   - Endarterectomy: Removal of atherosclerotic plaque from the arteries.
   - Vascular bypass: Restoration of blood flow by bypassing blocked vessels.
   - Thrombectomy: Removal of a blood clot from a vessel.

4. Thyroid and parathyroid gland surgery :
   - Thyroidectomy: partial or total removal of the thyroid gland.
   - Parathyroidectomy: removal of overactive parathyroid glands.

5. Colorectal surgery :
  - Colectomy: Removal of part of the colon.
  - Intestinal anastomosis: Connection of two intestinal segments.
  - Colorectal tumour resection: removal of tumours from the colon or rectum.

6. Hepatobiliary surgery :
  - Liver resection: removal of part of the liver.
  - Bile duct unblocking: Unblocking obstructed bile ducts.

7. Surgery of the upper digestive system :
  - Gastroplasty: Reduction in the size of the stomach to treat obesity.
  - Fundoplicature: Surgical repair of gastro-oesophageal reflux disease.

8. Bariatric surgery :
  - Gastric bypass: Creation of a short circuit in the stomach to reduce food absorption.

9. Endocrine surgery :
  - Adrenomectomy: removal of an adrenal gland.
  - Endocrine tumour resection: Removal of tumours of the endocrine glands.

10. Skin surgery :
  - Excision of skin tumours: Removal of skin tumours.
  - Skin grafts: Transplantation of skin for healing.

These areas of general surgery cover a wide range of medical conditions and surgical procedures. Each area requires specific skills and expertise to ensure safe and effective surgical outcomes.

Preparation for each type of general surgery varies according to the specifics of the procedure and the needs of the patient. However, there are some common elements to consider when preparing for different general surgeries. Here is an overview of specific preparation for some common types of general surgery:

1. Abdominal surgery (e.g. appendectomy, cholecystectomy) :
   - Preoperative fasting: The patient must refrain from eating and drinking in accordance with medical instructions.
   - Full pre-operative assessment: medical history, physical examinations, blood tests and imaging.
   - Skin preparation: The patient must shower with an antiseptic soap the day before surgery.

2. Thoracic surgery (e.g. pulmonary lobectomy) :
   - Pulmonary function tests: Pulmonary function tests may be carried out to assess lung capacity.
   - Prevention of pulmonary complications: Breathing and coughing exercises to reduce the risk of postoperative pulmonary complications.

3. Vascular surgery (e.g. endarterectomy, vascular bypass) :
   - Cardiac assessment: Cardiac tests may be required to assess the patient's heart health prior to surgery.
   - Vascular preparation: Examination of the blood vessels using imaging tests to plan the procedure.

4. Thyroid and parathyroid gland surgery :
   - Hormone check-up: Checking hormone levels to assess thyroid and parathyroid function.
   - Calcaemia assessment: To assess blood calcium levels in the event of parathyroid gland surgery.

5. Colorectal surgery (e.g. colectomy) :
   - Intestinal preparation: Elimination of faecal matter from the intestine before surgery using a special diet and laxatives.
   - Prophylactic antibiotic therapy: Administration of antibiotics prior to surgery to prevent infection.

6. Hepatobiliary surgery (e.g. liver resection) :
   - Liver function tests: Liver function tests to assess the liver's ability to recover after surgery.
   - Preparation for bleeding: Consider coagulation tests to ensure that coagulation function is optimal.

7. Surgery of the upper digestive system (e.g. gastroplasty) :
   - Nutritional assessment: Assessment of the patient's nutritional status prior to bariatric surgery.
   - Pre-operative training: Inform the patient about dietary changes and post-operative monitoring.

8. Obesity surgery (e.g. gastric bypass) :
   - Nutritional preparation: Follow a special diet before surgery to reduce the size of the liver and make the procedure easier.

9. Endocrine surgery (e.g. adrenomectomy) :
   - Hormone assessment: Assessment of hormone levels prior to surgery to guide post-operative management.

10. Skin surgery (e.g. removal of skin tumours) :
- Preparing the skin: Preparing the surgical area by cleansing and sterilising the skin.
It is important to note that each patient is unique and specific preparation may vary depending on individual factors. Preparation protocols are determined by the surgical team in consultation with the patient to ensure successful surgery and optimal recovery.

Orthopaedic surgery

Orthopaedic procedures are surgical interventions designed to diagnose, treat and correct musculoskeletal disorders. Here are some common orthopaedic procedures, including arthroplasty, fixation, fusion and others:

1. Arthroplasty (joint replacement) :
   - Hip replacement (total hip arthroplasty): Replacement of the hip joint with a metal and plastic prosthesis.
   - Knee replacement (total knee arthroplasty): Replacement of the knee joint with a prosthesis.
   - Shoulder arthroplasty: Replacement of the shoulder joint with a prosthesis.

2. Internal fixing :
   - Fracture repair: Use of screws, plates, nails and other devices to hold bones in place during healing.
   - Fixation of unstable joints: Use of devices to stabilise joints after injury or surgery.

3. Fusion (arthrodesis) :
   - Spinal arthrodesis: Fusion of vertebrae to treat spinal problems such as herniated discs or scoliosis.

- Arthrodesis of peripheral joints: Fusion of joints, such as the ankle or wrist, to treat severe arthritis.

4. Repair of tendons and ligaments :
   - Reconstruction of the anterior cruciate ligament (ACL): Reconstruction of the torn ACL using autogenous tissue or grafts.
   - Repair of torn tendons: Repair of tendons such as the Achilles tendon or shoulder tendons.

5. Nerve decompression :
   - Decompression of the median nerve (carpal tunnel syndrome): Release of the median nerve in the wrist to relieve pressure and pain.
   - Sciatic nerve decompression (discectomy): Removal of part of an intervertebral disc to relieve pressure on the sciatic nerve.

6. Osteotomy :
   - Hip osteotomy: surgical cutting of the bone to correct abnormalities in the hip joint.
   - Knee osteotomy: surgical correction of knee alignment to relieve joint pain.

7. Hand and foot surgery :
   - Carpal tunnel release: Relief of pressure on the median nerve in the wrist.
   - Correction of foot deformities: surgical correction of problems such as hallux valgus (bunion) or claw toes.

These common orthopaedic procedures illustrate the diversity of surgical interventions used to treat musculoskeletal disorders. Each procedure has its own specific indications, techniques and post-operative considerations, and they are all designed to improve patients' function and quality of life.

The handling of orthopaedic implants requires special care to ensure the success of the surgical procedure and the safety of the patient. Here are some important considerations for handling orthopaedic implants:

1. Safe storage and handling :
   - Implants must be stored in accordance with the manufacturer's recommendations to avoid contamination or damage.
   - Use strict precautions to avoid knocks, drops or any other handling that could damage the implants.

2. Traceability and identification :
   - Make sure that each implant is correctly labelled with precise information on type, size and batch number.
   - Check that the implants correspond to the specifications of the patient and the planned procedure.

3. Sterilisation :
   - Implants must be sterilised in accordance with established protocols to prevent post-operative infections.
   - Follow the manufacturer's sterilisation instructions to ensure effective sterilisation.

4. Handling techniques :
   - Use appropriate sterile instruments to handle the implants during surgery.
   - To avoid contamination, avoid touching critical parts of the implants with bare hands.

5. Integrity of packaging :
   - Only use implants whose packaging is intact and not compromised.
   - If the packaging is damaged, do not use the implant and report it in accordance with hospital protocols.

6. Precision and planning :
   - Follow the surgical plan carefully and ensure that the implants are correctly positioned in accordance with the plan.
   - Take into account the patient's anatomical specifications to ensure a precise fit.

7. Appropriate disposal :
   - Follow established protocols for the disposal of unused or expired implants in accordance with local regulations.

8. Training and awareness :
   - Surgical staff must be properly trained and aware of implant handling procedures.
   - Keep abreast of updates and ongoing training on new technologies and best practice.

9. Interdisciplinary communication :
   - Ensure effective communication between members of the surgical team to ensure that everyone is informed about the details of the procedure and the use of the implants.

By respecting these considerations and following the protocols established by the healthcare establishment and implant manufacturers, you will help to ensure the safety, effectiveness and success of orthopaedic surgery.

Cardiac surgery

Cardiac procedures are surgical interventions carried out to treat heart and vascular disorders. Here are some common types of cardiac procedures:
1. Coronary Artery Bypass Grafting (CABG) :

   - Blood vessels are taken from other parts of the body (such as the veins in the leg) to bypass the blocked coronary arteries, restoring blood flow to the heart.

2. Heart valve replacement or repair :
   - Aortic valve replacement: The defective aortic valve is replaced by a mechanical or biological valve.
   - Mitral valve replacement: The damaged mitral valve is replaced or repaired to restore normal blood circulation.

3. Aortic aneurysm surgery :
   - Abdominal aortic aneurysm repair: Repair of an enlarged area of the abdominal aorta using a synthetic graft.
   - Thoracic aortic aneurysm repair: Repair of the thoracic aorta with a synthetic graft.

4. Repair of atrial septal defect (ASD) or ventricular septal defect (VSD) :
   - Closing abnormal openings between the heart chambers to prevent circulatory problems.

149

5. Surgery for atrial fibrillation :
   - Surgical removal of the heart tissue responsible for arrhythmias to restore a regular heart rhythm.

6. Heart transplantation :
   - Replacement of the damaged heart with a healthy heart from a compatible donor.

7. Endocarditis surgery :
   - Repair or replacement of heart valves damaged by bacterial infection.

8. Surgery for aortic stenosis :
   - Repair or replacement of the narrowed aortic valve to improve blood flow.

9. Repair of tetralogy of Fallot :
   - Repair of congenital heart defects, including correction of ventricular septal defects and restoration of normal blood flow.

10. Surgery for aortic dissection :
   - Repair of a tear in the aortic wall to prevent serious complications.

These cardiac procedures are performed to treat a range of cardiac disorders, whether congenital, acquired or age-related. Each procedure has its own specific indications, techniques and considerations, and they are all designed to restore or improve the patient's cardiac function and quality of life.

Advanced monitoring and management of specific risk factors is essential to ensure positive outcomes in complex surgical procedures and to minimise complications. Here are some important considerations for monitoring and managing specific risk factors in the surgical setting:

1. Haemodynamic monitoring :
   - Continuous monitoring of blood pressure, heart rate and oxygen saturation to detect haemodynamic changes.

2. Electrocardiogram (ECG) monitoring :
   - Monitoring of the heart's electrical activity to detect arrhythmias or signs of cardiac ischaemia.

3. Blood glucose management :
   - Monitoring and maintaining blood glucose levels within appropriate limits to avoid metabolic complications.

4. Fluid management and electrolyte balance :
   - Continuous assessment of fluid and electrolyte balance to prevent dehydration and electrolyte imbalances.

5. Prevention of deep vein thrombosis (DVT) :
   - Use of intermittent pneumatic compression devices and anticoagulants to prevent DVT and pulmonary embolism.

6. Infection prevention :
   - Use of prophylactic antibiotics before surgery to reduce the risk of post-operative infections.

7. Ventilation monitoring :
   - Assessment of lung function, monitoring of respiratory rate and oxygen saturation to detect respiratory problems.

8. Pain management :
   - Use of analgesics and pain management techniques to ensure patient comfort and promote rapid recovery.

9. Prevention of thromboembolic complications :
   - Use of anticoagulants, compression stockings and early mobilisation to prevent blood clots.

10. Neurological monitoring :
   - Assessment of neurological function to detect any signs of neurological deficits, such as confusion or weakness.

11. Management of anaemia :
   - Management of pre-operative and post-operative anaemia to avoid complications associated with low haemoglobin levels.

12. Hypothermia management :
   - Maintaining the patient's body temperature to avoid hypothermia, which can increase the risk of complications.

13. Prevention of urinary retention :
   • Monitoring diuresis and implementing measures to prevent urinary retention.

14. Nutrition management :
   • Ensure adequate nutrition to support post-operative healing and recovery.

Advanced monitoring and proactive management of these specific risk factors require close coordination between members of the surgical team and well-established protocols. A multidisciplinary approach and effective communication are essential to optimise surgical outcomes and minimise post-operative complications.

Neurological surgery

Neurosurgical interventions are surgical procedures performed on the central and peripheral nervous system to diagnose, treat or relieve neurological disorders. Here are some common types of neurosurgical procedures:

1. Tumorectomy :
   • Surgical removal of a brain or spinal tumour to reduce pressure on surrounding tissue and treat associated symptoms.

2. Decompression :
   • Decompression of the spinal cord or nerves to relieve compression due to herniated discs, tumours or other abnormalities.

3. Deep brain stimulation (DBS) :
   • Implanting electrodes in specific areas of the brain to treat neurological disorders such as Parkinson's disease, essential tremor or dystonia.
4. Craniotomy :
   • Surgical opening of the skull to access the brain and treat various conditions, including trauma, aneurysms and vascular malformations.

5. Resection of epilepsy :
   - Surgical removal of the area of the brain responsible for epileptic seizures to reduce the frequency and severity of seizures.

6. Cerebral aneurysm surgery :
   - Repair of aneurysms (abnormal dilations of blood vessels) in the brain to prevent rupture and bleeding.

7. Vascular malformation surgery :
   - Repair of arteriovenous malformations (AVMs) or capillary malformations to prevent bleeding and complications.

8. Spinal surgery :
   - Intervention on the spinal column to treat conditions such as herniated discs, spinal stenosis or spinal deformities.

9. Functional surgery :
   - Interventions to treat movement disorders, such as Parkinson's disease or dystonia, by modifying the neuronal circuits responsible.

10. Pain surgery :
    - Intervention to treat chronic pain by cutting or modifying the nerves involved in pain transmission.

11. Peripheral nerve surgery :
    - Repair of nerve damage, tumours or inflammation affecting peripheral nerves.

These neurosurgical procedures require specialist expertise and close coordination between the surgical team and other healthcare professionals. Each procedure has specific indications and unique post-operative considerations to ensure patient recovery and quality of life.

Maintaining a sterile environment in neurosurgical procedures, particularly brain surgery, is crucial to reducing the risk of postoperative infections and ensuring patient safety. Here are some key techniques for maintaining a sterile environment during these delicate procedures:

1. Careful preparation of the operating theatre :
   - The operating theatre must be thoroughly cleaned and disinfected before surgery.
   - Use of sterile covers to cover non-essential surfaces, equipment and furniture.

2. Appropriate washing and dressing :
   - The surgical team must follow strict protocols for washing hands and dressing in sterile surgical garments.
   - Use of masks, caps, goggles and sterile gloves to minimise the spread of particles.

3. Installation of sterile fields :
   - Use of sterile drapes to cover the incision area, instruments and instrument tables.
   - The fields are handled with care to avoid contamination.

4. Use of barriers and adhesive sheets :
   - Use of protective barriers such as adhesive sheets to demarcate sterile and non-sterile areas.
   - These barriers prevent the migration of bacteria and maintain sterility.

5. Aseptic handling of instruments :
   - Use of sterile instruments and aseptic handling throughout the procedure.
   - Instruments are placed on sterile drapes and handled with sterile forceps to avoid contamination.

6. Environmental control :
   - Reduced air circulation in the operating theatre to minimise particle dispersion.
   - Use of HEPA air filtration systems to maintain a clean atmosphere.

7. Limiting non-essential movements :
   - Non-essential movements in the operating theatre are kept to a minimum to avoid air turbulence.

8. Preventing splashes and spills :
   - Prevent splashes of body fluids by using sterile drapes and avoiding sudden movements.
   - Use of absorbent pads to collect fluids during the procedure.

9. Continuous sterility monitoring :
   - A dedicated person constantly monitors compliance with sterility protocols during surgery.
   - Any breach of sterility is immediately reported and rectified.

These techniques are crucial to creating and maintaining a sterile environment during brain surgery and other neurosurgical procedures. Communication and vigilance on the part of the surgical team are essential to ensure compliance with protocols and patient safety.

Gynecologygical and obstetric surgery

Gynecologygical surgery encompasses a wide range of surgical procedures performed on the female reproductive system. Here are some examples of common gynecologygical surgeries:

1. Hysterectomy :
   - Surgical removal of the uterus, sometimes together with the ovaries and fallopian tubes.
   - Indicated for a variety of conditions, including fibroids, endometriosis, abnormal uterine bleeding and uterine cancer.

2. Cystectomy :
   - Surgical removal of the bladder, sometimes necessary to treat bladder cancer or other serious conditions.

3. Urinary incontinence surgery :
   - Repair of the supporting tissues of the bladder and urethra to treat urinary incontinence.

4. Pelvic prolapse surgery :
   - Repair of pelvic organs that have slipped from their normal position, such as the uterus, bladder or rectum.

5. Myomectomy :
   - Surgical removal of uterine fibroids while preserving the uterus for women who wish to retain their fertility.

6. Surgery for endometriosis :
   - Removal of endometrial tissue that develops outside the uterus and causes pain and complications.

7. Surgery for fertility disorders :
   - Repair of anatomical anomalies that can affect fertility, such as polyps, adhesions or obstructions.

8. Surgery for gynecologygical cancer :
   - Surgery to treat cancers of the cervix, ovary, uterus, vagina and vulva.

9. Tubal ligation (tubal sterilisation) :
   - Procedure to prevent fertilisation by blocking or cutting the fallopian tubes.

10. Biopsies and excisions :
   - Tissue sampling for the diagnosis or treatment of various gynecologygical conditions.

Each type of gynecologygical surgery has its own indications, techniques and post-operative considerations. The aim of these procedures is to improve women's gynecologygical health, treat medical conditions and preserve fertility where possible. Technological advances and minimally invasive surgical approaches have also helped to improve outcomes and recovery for many patients.

Support during caesarean sections and other obstetric procedures is essential to support patients and ensure positive medical and psychological outcomes. Here's how support can be provided during these procedures:

1. Preoperative information :
   - Before the caesarean section or any other obstetric procedure, the medical team must explain to the patient what the procedure involves, why she needs it and the steps to be taken.
   - The risks, benefits and alternatives must be discussed to enable the patient to make an informed decision.

2. Emotional support :
   - Obstetric operations can be stressful for patients. Healthcare professionals and relatives must be on hand to provide emotional support, reassurance and answer patients' questions.
   - The presence of a partner, family member or doula can help reduce anxiety.

3. Open communication :
   - The medical team must maintain open communication with the patient throughout the process. Explaining each step as it unfolds can help reduce uncertainty.

4. Anaesthesia and comfort :
   - If an anaesthetic is used, explanations of how it works and what to expect are essential.
   - Ensure the patient's comfort by positioning her body correctly and taking precautions to avoid any pain.

5. Active participation :
   - Whenever possible and safe, involve the patient in the process. For example, she may be allowed to touch or hold her baby whenever appropriate.

6. Explain the events and results :
   - As the procedure progresses, healthcare professionals should explain what is happening, the next steps and the results.

7. Post-operative care and recovery :
   - Once the procedure is complete, medical follow-up and post-operative care are essential to monitor the recovery of the patient and baby.

8. Psychological support :
   - After the procedure, provide psychological support to help the patient cope with the emotions and feelings that may arise.

9. Postoperative education :
   - Provide the patient with information on home care, precautions and signs to look out for.

Support during caesarean sections and other obstetric procedures aims to create a positive and respectful experience for the patient, while ensuring her safety and that of her baby. Empathetic communication and a patient-centred care environment are key elements of this support.

Urological surgery

Urological procedures refer to a range of surgeries performed on the urinary system, including the kidneys, bladder, prostate, urethra and other associated organs. Here are some examples of common urological procedures:

1. Prostatectomy :
   - Total or partial surgical removal of the prostate, usually to treat prostate cancer.
   - Various surgical approaches can be used, including open, laparoscopic or robot-assisted prostatectomy.

2. Nephrectomy :
   - Surgical removal of a kidney, either partially (partial nephrectomy) or completely (total nephrectomy).
   - Indicated for treating kidney cancer, renal cysts, trauma or living kidney donors.
   -

3. Cystectomy :
   - Surgical removal of the bladder, usually to treat bladder cancer.
   - This often involves the creation of a new urine outlet (ileal conduit or neo-bladder).

4. Urinary incontinence surgery :
   - Repair of the supporting tissues of the bladder and urethra to treat urinary incontinence.

5. Lithotripsy :
   - Use of shock waves to break up kidney or ureter stones into small pieces, facilitating their removal.

6. Transurethral resection of the prostate (TURP) :
   - Removal of parts of the prostate through the urethra to treat benign prostatic hypertrophy.

7. Urethra surgery :
   - Surgical repair of the urethra to treat problems such as narrowing or trauma.

8. Urological reconstructive surgery :
   - Surgical repair of the urinary tract to treat congenital anomalies, trauma or malformations.

9. Bladder reconstruction surgery :
   - Creation of a new bladder from other parts of the body after a cystectomy.

10. Renal transplant surgery :
   - Transplantation of a kidney from a living or deceased donor into a patient suffering from renal failure.

These procedures are designed to treat a variety of urological conditions and improve patients' health and quality of life. Technological advances, such as robot-assisted surgery, have also improved surgical results and post-operative recovery.

Specific preparation for endoscopic urological procedures plays a crucial role in the success of the operation and in reducing the risks to the patient. The following are typical steps in preparation for such procedures:

1. Medical assessment :
   - The medical team assesses the patient's overall health, including medical history, allergies and current medication.
   - Pre-operative tests such as blood tests, electrocardiogram (ECG) and renal function assessments can be carried out.

2. Information and informed consent :
   - The patient receives detailed information about the procedure, the risks, the benefits and possible alternatives.
   - The patient must give informed consent for the procedure.

3. Fasting :
   - The patient is informed of the fasting instructions (food and fluids) before the procedure.
   - Fasting is essential to reduce the risk of complications associated with anaesthesia.

4. Intestinal preparation :
   - For some procedures, it may be necessary to prepare the intestines by taking medication to empty the intestinal contents (laxatives).

5. Medicines :
   - Medications can be adjusted or temporarily stopped before the procedure, particularly anticoagulants, non-steroidal anti-inflammatory drugs (NSAIDs) and agents that affect coagulation.

6. Personal hygiene :
   - The patient is informed of the importance of good personal hygiene, including cleaning the genital area.

7. Arrival at the hospital :
   - The patient reports to the hospital in accordance with the instructions provided.

8. Preparing the operating theatre :
   - The operating theatre is prepared with the instruments, equipment and devices required for the endoscopic procedure.

9. Anaesthesia :
   - Local, regional or general anaesthesia may be administered depending on the procedure and the patient's needs.

10. Positioning the patient :
   - The patient is positioned to allow optimum access to the target area for the endoscopic procedure.

11. Sterilisation and asepsis :
   - The medical team follows strict safety protocols.
   - This is the first time that a patient has undergone sterilisation and asepsis to reduce the risk of infection.

12. Endoscopic procedure :
   - The endoscopic procedure is carried out in accordance with the techniques specific to each operation.

Adequate preparation helps to minimise risks and ensure that the endoscopic urological procedure goes smoothly.

Communication between the patient and the medical team is essential to ensure that all instructions are followed and that the patient is ready for the procedure.

Plastic and reconstructive surgery

Aesthetic and reconstructive surgery techniques encompass a wide range of procedures aimed at improving physical appearance or restoring functionality after injury, congenital deformity or previous surgery. Here are some examples of cosmetic and reconstructive surgery techniques:

1. Facelift :
   - Removal of excess skin and underlying tissue to rejuvenate the appearance of the face and neck.
   - Different variations include the forehead lift, the cervico-facial lift and the mini-lift.

2. Rhinoplasty :
   - Nose surgery to modify its size, shape or functionality.
   - May involve reducing, increasing or correcting deformations.

3. Breast reconstruction :
   - Restoration of the breast after a mastectomy or loss of breast tissue.
   - Use of breast implants or autologous tissue (flap).

4. Breast augmentation :
   - Surgery to increase the size of the breasts using breast implants or lipofilling (fat transfer).

5. Breast reduction :
   - Reduction in breast size to relieve physical discomfort and improve body proportion.

6. Liposuction :
   - Surgical removal of localised fat deposits to reshape body contours.

7. Abdominoplasty (tummy tuck) :
   - Removal of excess skin and fat from the abdomen for a flatter, more toned tummy.

8. Eyelid surgery (blepharoplasty) :
   • Reduction of excess skin and fat around the eyes to rejuvenate appearance and improve visibility.

9. Lip and chin surgery :
   • Augmentation or reduction of the lips and chin to improve facial proportions.

10. Reconstructive limb surgery :
   • Repairs to injuries, deformities or deformities of the arms, legs, hands or feet.

These cosmetic and reconstructive surgery techniques are performed by qualified and experienced surgeons. For aesthetic procedures, a thorough consultation with the patient is essential to discuss goals, expectations and potential risks. For reconstructive procedures, the aim is to restore functionality and natural appearance as far as possible. Technological advances and minimally invasive surgical approaches have also played an important role in improving patient outcomes and recovery.

Preparation for tissue grafting and microsurgery is a detailed process designed to ensure the success of the procedure and the health of the patient. The following are typical steps in preparing for such complex procedures:

1. Full medical assessment :
   • A thorough assessment of the patient's general health is carried out, including medical history, allergies, medication and pre-operative examinations.

2. Consultation and planning :
   • A detailed consultation with the surgeon is necessary to discuss the objectives of the graft or microsurgery, the patient's expectations and the options available.
   • The procedure is carefully planned, including the choice of donor and recipient sites.

3. Preparing the patient :
   • The patient is given information about the procedure, the risks, the benefits and the possible outcomes.
   • The patient must understand the post-operative requirements and agree to follow the instructions.

4. Preparation of the donor site :
   - If the procedure requires tissue or a graft to be taken from another part of the patient's body, the donor site is carefully prepared.

5. Preoperative marking :
   - The surgeon can mark the recipient and donor sites on the patient's body to guide the procedure.

6. Anaesthesia :
   - The type of anaesthetic (local, regional or general) is determined according to the procedure and the patient's needs.

7. Sterilisation and asepsis :
   - Sterilisation of the operating theatre and preparation of instruments are essential to minimise the risk of infection.

8. Advanced microsurgery :
   - Surgeons use microscopes and high-precision instruments to perform anastomoses (blood vessel connections) and to graft tissue.

9. Continuous monitoring :
   - During the procedure, the patient is constantly monitored to ensure that the graft is successful and that blood circulation is adequate.

10. Specific post-operative care :
   - The patient receives detailed instructions for post-operative care, including pain management, dressings and medication.

11. Medical follow-up :
   - Follow-up visits are planned to monitor healing, assess the vascularisation of the graft and adjust treatments if necessary.

Tissue grafting and microsurgery procedures require advanced surgical expertise and rigorous preparation to achieve successful results. Close collaboration between the surgeon, anaesthetist and care team is essential to ensure patient safety and a successful procedure.

Paediatric surgery

Paediatric surgery presents specific considerations due to the anatomical, physiological and psychological differences between children and adults. Here are some of the key considerations for paediatric surgery:

1. Instrument sizes :
   - Surgical instruments must be adapted to the size of the patient, taking into account anatomical differences in children.
   - Miniaturised instruments may be required for infants and young children.

2. Dosage of medicines :
   - Drug doses should be adjusted according to the child's weight, age and metabolism.
   - Accurate dose calculation is crucial to avoid over- or under-dosing.

3. Anaesthesia :
   - Paediatric anaesthesia requires special expertise, as children may react differently to anaesthetic agents.
   - Regional anaesthesia techniques (epidural, spinal) may be preferred for some children.

4. Post-operative care :
   - Children may have different recovery needs, requiring careful monitoring of breathing, pain and circulation.
   - Pain management must be adapted to the child's age and preferences.

5. Communication and psychology :
   - Children have specific psychological needs. It is important to reassure them and explain the procedure in a way that is adapted to their level of understanding.
   - The use of distraction and play techniques can reduce anxiety and facilitate cooperation.

6. Surgery on neonates and premature babies :
   - Premature babies or babies born with health problems require special surgical and anaesthetic care.

7. Nutrition and hydration :
   - Children's nutritional and water requirements differ from those of adults. It is important to maintain an adequate balance during the perioperative period.

8. Outpatient surgery :
   - Outpatient paediatric surgery requires careful planning to ensure safe and rapid recovery at home.

9. Specialised equipment :
   - Some special equipment, such as catheters and safety devices, may be needed to adapt to children.

10. Ethics and consent :
   - Informed consent from parents or legal guardians is essential for paediatric interventions. Decision-making must be ethical and respectful.

Paediatric surgery requires a multidisciplinary approach, involving paediatric surgeons, paediatric anaesthetists, paediatric nurses and other healthcare professionals. Particular attention to considerations specific to children ensures optimal surgical results and minimises potential risks.

Preparing children and their families emotionally before surgery is essential to reduce anxiety, encourage cooperation and improve the overall outcome of the procedure. Here are some approaches to preparing children and their families emotionally:

1. Age-appropriate communication :
   - Explain the procedure in a simple, age-appropriate way. Use familiar words and concrete examples.

2. Preoperative visit :
   - Organise a preoperative tour of the operating theatre so that the child can see the environment and ask questions.

3. Books and videos :
   - Use books and videos designed to explain surgery and the hospital process in a fun and understandable way.

4. Role play :
   - Use dolls or stuffed animals to simulate the procedure and show what will happen.

5. Distraction tools :
   - Provide toys, books or tablets to distract the child before the procedure.

6. Listening and answering questions :
   - Encourage the child to ask questions and answer them honestly. Reassure them of the normal sensations they may experience.

7. Involving parents :
   - Involve parents actively in the preparation process and encourage them to ask questions and share their concerns.

8. Emotional support :
   - Offer emotional support by reassuring the child that the doctors and nurses are there to protect him or her.

9. Family integration :
   - Involve the family in the preparation process to increase emotional support and reduce anxiety.

10. Use of visual aids :
   - Show photos or videos of children preparing for surgery and then recovering.

11. Respect for individual needs :
   - Every child reacts differently to emotional preparation. Be attentive to their specific needs.

12. Support during the process :
   - Make sure that a family member can accompany the child to the operating theatre and meet him or her after the operation.

13. Post-operative follow-up :
   - Offer ongoing support and provide information on recovery and post-operative care.

Preparing children and their families emotionally is an important part of paediatric care. By reducing anxiety and providing clear information, you help to create a reassuring environment conducive to a positive experience for the child and his or her family.

Outpatient surgery

Managing outpatient surgical procedures, also known as ambulatory or outpatient surgery, requires careful planning and a specific approach to ensure patient safety and well-being. Here are the key steps in managing outpatient surgery:

1. Preoperative assessment :
   * Patients must undergo a full medical assessment to ensure they are suitable for outpatient surgery.
   * Medical history, allergies, medication and pre-existing conditions are examined.

2. Planning the procedure :
   * Appropriate choice of surgical procedure based on outpatient feasibility and expected recovery.
   * Determining the equipment, personnel and resources required.

3. Informed consent :
   * Patients need to understand the benefits, risks and alternatives of outpatient surgery.
   * Informed consent must be obtained in accordance with ethical protocols.

4. Preparing the patient :
   * Patients receive detailed instructions on pre-operative preparation, including fasting, medication and skin care.

5. Anaesthesia :
   * Anaesthesia is chosen according to the procedure and the patient's needs. Local, regional or general anaesthesia may be used.

6. Surgery :
- The surgical procedure is carried out with precision and attention to detail.
- Asepsis and sterilisation protocols are scrupulously followed to prevent infections.

7. Postoperative recovery :
- Patients are carefully monitored in a recovery room until they are stable and awake.
- Pain is managed and patients are prepared to return home.

8. Patient and carer education :
- Patients and their carers are given specific instructions on post-operative care, the signs to look out for and who to contact if they have any concerns.

9. Post-operative follow-up :
- Follow-up appointments are scheduled to assess the patient's healing and recovery.

10. Management of complications :
- Patients receive information on how to manage potential complications, such as excessive bleeding or infection.

11. Ongoing communication :
- Communication between the medical team, patients and carers is essential to ensure a smooth recovery.

12. Access to emergency care :
- Patients must be informed of the measures to be taken in the event of a serious complication after discharge.

13. Quality monitoring and assessment :
- The medical team regularly evaluates ambulatory surgery protocols and implements improvements where necessary.

The management of outpatient surgery aims to provide high-quality care in a safe and comfortable environment. Open communication, well-defined protocols and careful planning help to ensure the success of these procedures and patient satisfaction.

Patient preparation and post-operative monitoring for same-day discharges, also known as ambulatory or outpatient surgery, are essential steps in ensuring the safety and recovery of patients following surgery. Here are the key steps in the preparation and post-operative monitoring of same-day discharges:

Preparing the patient :
1. Preoperative assessment :
   - Patients undergo a thorough medical assessment to ensure they are eligible for same-day discharge.
   - Medical history, allergies, current medication and pre-existing conditions are assessed.

2. Preoperative education :
   - Patients receive detailed information about the procedure, post-operative care, signs of complications and what to do if they need to.

3. Preparing at home :
   - Patients receive specific instructions on fasting, pre-operative medication and skin care before surgery.

4. Informed consent :
   - Patients understand the details of the surgery, the associated risks and give their informed consent in accordance with ethical protocols.

Post-operative monitoring :
1. Recovery room :
   - Patients are carefully monitored in a recovery room until they are awake, stable and their vital signs are normal.

2. Pain management :
   - Patients are given appropriate analgesic medication to manage postoperative pain.

3. Recovery and responsiveness :
   - The team monitors signs of recovery and checks the patient's responsiveness after anaesthesia.

4. Assessment of vital signs :
   - Vital signs such as blood pressure, heart rate, respiratory rate and oxygen saturation are monitored regularly.

5. Checking wounds and drains :
   - Dressings, drains and surgical incisions are checked for signs of infection, excessive bleeding or problems.

6. Exit evaluation :
   - Specific discharge criteria are assessed, such as haemodynamic stability and the ability to drink, urinate and walk.

7. Postoperative education :
   - Patients and their carers receive detailed instructions on post-operative care at home, the medication to be taken and the signs of complications.

8. Post-exit follow-up :
   - Patients receive a follow-up telephone call or appointment to assess their recovery and resolve any concerns.

Patient preparation and post-operative monitoring for same-day discharges aim to ensure a safe and effective recovery from outpatient surgery. Clear communication between the medical team, the patient and their carers is crucial to ensure that the patient is well informed and ready to manage the first days of recovery at home.

Chapter 7:
Instrument and equipment management

Importance of efficient management of instruments and equipment

Proper preparation of surgical instruments has a significant impact on patient safety throughout the surgical procedure. Careful and rigorous instrument preparation helps to reduce the risk of infections, complications and medical errors, ensuring a safe and optimal surgical environment for the patient. Here's how proper instrument preparation affects patient safety:

1. Infection prevention :
   - Effective instrument sterilisation eliminates potentially pathogenic micro-organisms, significantly reducing the risk of post-operative infections.

2. Reducing complications :
   - Properly prepared instruments minimise the risk of complications such as excessive bleeding, wound infections and adverse reactions.

3. Surgical precision :
   - Sharp, ready-to-use instruments allow surgeons to make more precise incisions and sutures, improving surgical outcomes.

4. Avoid delays :
   - Proper instrument preparation ensures that the necessary equipment is available immediately, avoiding delays during the procedure.

5. Minimising errors :
   - The steps involved in preparing and checking instruments help to reduce medical errors linked to the use of incorrect or badly prepared instruments.

6. Smooth procedure :
  • When the instruments are ready and well organised, the surgical procedure runs smoothly, which can reduce the length of the operation and the stress for the team and the patient.

7. Compliance with safety standards :
  • Proper instrument preparation is essential to meet strict sterilisation and asepsis standards, ensuring a safe surgical environment.

8. Post-operative management :
  • Successful surgery thanks to proper instrument preparation can have a positive impact on the patient's recovery period and recovery.

9. Team confidence :
  • When the surgical team knows that the instruments are correctly prepared, it increases confidence in the process and encourages smooth collaboration.

10. Patient satisfaction :
  • An uncomplicated surgical procedure using appropriately prepared instruments can contribute to patient satisfaction and a successful recovery.

In summary, proper preparation of surgical instruments is an essential component of patient safety. It plays a major role in reducing risks, improving surgical outcomes and ensuring a safe and effective surgical environment for all patients.

The nurse's role in ensuring the functionality of equipment is crucial to the safety and success of surgical procedures. Medical and surgical equipment plays an essential role in carrying out an effective and safe surgical procedure, and it is the nurse's responsibility to ensure that this equipment is in perfect working order. Here's how the nurse contributes to ensuring the functionality of the equipment:

1. Preoperative check :
  • Before the start of each surgical procedure, the nurse carries out a thorough check of all the necessary equipment. This includes surgical instruments, vital sign

monitors, anaesthesia machines, lighting and operating tables.

2. Calibration and testing :
   - The nurse ensures that the equipment is correctly calibrated and tested to guarantee its accuracy. This includes checking parameters such as pressure, temperature and heart rate.

3. Preparing the equipment :
   - Before surgery, the nurse prepares all the necessary equipment and places it within easy reach of the surgeon and surgical team.

4. Preventive maintenance :
   - The nurse takes part in regular preventive maintenance activities, such as cleaning, lubricating and servicing equipment, to avoid unexpected breakdowns.

5. Identifying problems :
   - If any equipment malfunctions or shows signs of failure, the nurse immediately reports the problem to the maintenance team or the designated manager.

6. Emergency response :
   - In the event of an emergency or equipment failure during a procedure, the nurse must be able to take rapid action to resolve the problem and ensure the continuity of the surgery.

7. Interdisciplinary collaboration :
   - The nurse works closely with biomedical technicians, biomedical engineers and other members of the healthcare team to ensure that equipment is properly maintained and repaired.

8. Further training :
   - Nurses take part in ongoing training programmes on the use, maintenance and safety of medical equipment to keep up to date with the latest practices and technologies.

9. Documentation :
- The nurse keeps precise records of checks, tests and interventions carried out on equipment, ensuring traceability and transparency.

The nurse's role in ensuring the functionality of equipment is essential to creating a safe and effective surgical environment. By working closely with the medical and maintenance teams, nurses help to minimise the risk of equipment malfunctions, ensure quality of care and improve surgical outcomes for patients.

Identification and organisation of surgical instruments

Surgical instruments are classified into different categories according to their specific use in the surgical context. Each category of instrument has a specific role in the performance of surgical procedures. The following is a common classification of instruments according to their use:

1. Dissecting instruments :
- These instruments are used to cut, separate and remove tissue during surgery. Examples: scalpels, dissecting scissors, lifts.

2. Tools for gripping and holding :
- These instruments are used to grasp, hold and manipulate tissues and organs during surgery. Examples: anatomical forceps, Kocher forceps, grasping forceps.

3. Shrinking tools :
- These instruments are designed to hold the tissues apart, providing better visibility of the surgical site. Examples: Farabeuf retractors, Cushing retractors.

4. Suture and anastomosis instruments :
- They are used to make sutures and stitches, as well as to anastomose (connect) tissues. Examples: suture needles, needle holders, suture forceps.

5. Coagulation and haemostasis instruments :
   - These instruments are used to control bleeding by cauterising blood vessels. Examples: haemostatic forceps, electric scalpel, bipolar coagulator.

6. Suction and irrigation instruments :
   - Used to remove fluids and debris from the surgical site, and to irrigate and clean the area. Examples: suction cannulas, irrigation syringes.

7. Measuring instruments :
   - They are used to measure the dimensions and depths of tissue, and to assess distances during specific procedures. Examples: surgical rulers, calipers.

8. Reconstruction tools :
   - These instruments are used for tissue reconstruction, implant fixation or the creation of anatomical shapes. Examples: surgical stapler, osteosynthesis equipment.

9. Instruments specific to surgery :
   - Some instruments are specific to a particular type of surgery, such as orthopaedic, ophthalmic, gynecologygical and neurosurgical instruments.
10. Measurement and assessment tools :
   - Used to assess organ function, blood circulation or other physiological parameters. Examples: Doppler, blood pressure monitor, pulse oximeter.

It is important to note that this classification is not exhaustive and that new instruments may be developed in line with technological advances and clinical needs. Each instrument has a specific role in the surgical process and requires expert handling by the surgical team to ensure patient safety and the success of the procedure.

During surgery, efficient organisation and appropriate sorting of instruments, equipment and supplies are essential to ensure a smooth and rapid recovery. Here are some sorting and organising techniques that can help to improve workflow in the operating theatre:

1. Sorted by use :
   - Sort instruments and equipment according to their specific use in the surgical procedure. This allows you to quickly locate what you need at each stage of the operation.

2. Prepared trays :
   - Prepare trays of pre-assembled instruments according to the stages of the surgery. Each tray should contain the instruments needed for a specific part of the procedure.

3. Spatial organisation :
   - Arrange the instruments and equipment logically on the operating table, placing the necessary items within easy reach of the surgeon and assistants.

4. Use of preparation bags :
   - Use sterile bags or envelopes to group similar instruments. This helps maintain asepsis while facilitating access to the necessary tools.

5. Clear labelling :
   - Label trays, bags and containers clearly and legibly to quickly identify their contents.

6. Preoperative communication :
   - Discuss the surgical plan with the team before the procedure to clarify instrument and material requirements at each stage.

7. Team preparation :
   - Involve all members of the surgical team in the preparation and organisation of the equipment to ensure better coordination.

8. Quick removal of unused instruments :
   - Remove unused instruments from the work area immediately to avoid clutter and allow the team to concentrate on the tasks in hand.

9. Continuous monitoring :
   - The circulating nurse monitors the use of instruments and equipment, quickly replaces depleted items and ensures that everything is ready for the next step.

10. Avoid redundancies :
  • Limit the number of similar instruments on the operating table to avoid confusion and clutter.

11. Use of digital dashboards :
  • Use touch screens or digital dashboards to display essential information about instruments, the stages of surgery and the patient's vital signs.

12. Reassessment during the procedure :
  • Reassess instrument and material requirements regularly as surgery progresses, and adjust the organisation accordingly.

Efficient organisation in the operating theatre helps to reduce operating time, minimise errors and delays, and ensure rapid and safe patient recovery. By adopting these triage and organisation techniques, the surgical team can improve coordination, communication and safety during surgery.

Instrument preparation and quality control

Cleaning, disinfection and visual inspection of surgical instruments are crucial steps in maintaining asepsis, preventing infection and ensuring patient safety. Here's an overview of these essential processes:

1. Cleaning :
  • Initial cleaning aims to remove organic debris, body fluids and tissue residues from instruments. It can include steps such as pre-soaking, manual brushing and the use of ultrasound. Cleaning is often the first step in preparing instruments for further disinfection.

2. Disinfection :
  • After cleaning, instruments undergo disinfection to eliminate potentially pathogenic micro-organisms. There are various methods of disinfection, including chemical disinfection and thermal disinfection. Some instruments may undergo sterilisation after disinfection to achieve a high level of asepsis.

3. Visual inspection :
  • A thorough visual inspection is carried out after cleaning and disinfection to detect any residue, damage or signs of wear on the instruments. This helps to identify instruments that require repair, replacement or an additional cleaning step.

4. Use of magnifiers and lighting :
  • Magnifying glasses and appropriate lighting are used during the visual inspection to detect residual particles or minor problems that may not be visible to the naked eye.

5. Documentation :
  • Each stage of the cleaning, disinfection and visual inspection process is carefully documented to ensure traceability and compliance with safety standards.

6. Corrosion prevention :
  • Stainless steel instruments must be dried properly after cleaning and disinfection to prevent corrosion. The use of appropriate drying agents is important.

7. Repair and replacement :
  • Instruments that are damaged or show signs of excessive wear are repaired or replaced according to established protocols. Instruments must be in perfect working order before being used again.

8. Quality control :
  • The cleaning, disinfection and inspection processes are subject to regular quality controls to ensure that they are effective and comply with standards.

It is essential that the surgical team, including nurses and sterilisation technicians, strictly follow established protocols for cleaning, disinfecting and inspecting instruments. These steps are essential for maintaining a sterile and safe environment in the operating theatre, minimising the risk of nosocomial infections and ensuring optimal surgical results.

The use of autoclaves and other sterilisation equipment is a crucial step in the preparation of surgical instruments and equipment to ensure a sterile environment in the operating theatre. Here's how this equipment is used in the sterilisation process:

1. Autoclaves :

- Autoclaves are pressurised steam sterilisation devices. They are used to destroy pathogenic micro-organisms present on surgical instruments. Here are the typical steps involved in using autoclaves:

- Loading: Clean and prepared instruments are placed in trays, bags or containers suitable for sterilisation.

- Programming: The sterilisation cycle is chosen according to the type of instruments and materials used.

- Preheating: The autoclave is preheated to the required temperature and pressure.

- Sterilisation: Instruments are exposed to pressurised steam for a set period of time. The high temperature and steam eliminate micro-organisms.

- Cooling: Once sterilisation is complete, the instruments are cooled before being removed from the autoclave.

2. Other sterilisation methods :

- In addition to autoclaves, other sterilisation methods include :

- Ethylene oxide sterilisation: This gas is used to sterilise instruments that are sensitive to heat and humidity.

- Radiation sterilisation: Instruments are exposed to gamma rays or X-rays to destroy micro-organisms.

- Chemical sterilisation: Chemical agents are used to sterilise heat-sensitive instruments.

179

3. Sterility check :
  - Once the sterilisation process is complete, autoclaves and other devices are fitted with monitoring systems and chemical indicators to check that sterilisation has been carried out successfully. Biological and chemical tests are also used periodically to validate the effectiveness of the sterilisation process.

4. Handling after sterilisation :
  - Sterilised instruments must be handled with care to avoid contamination. They are stored in specific areas and in sterile packaging until they are used in the operating theatre.

5. Monitoring and documentation :
  - All stages of the sterilisation process, including sterilisation parameters, test results and sterility shelf life, are meticulously documented to ensure traceability and compliance with standards.

The appropriate use of autoclaves and other sterilisation devices is essential to maintain a safe and sterile surgical environment. Healthcare professionals must be trained in sterilisation protocols, the handling of sterilised instruments and follow-up procedures to ensure high-quality care and prevent nosocomial infections.

Management of implants and medical devices

Safe storage and traceability of surgical implants are critical aspects of instrument and material management in the operating theatre. Here's how to ensure effective management of these implants:

1. Safe storage :
  - Surgical implants must be stored in specific, controlled environments to prevent contamination or damage. Measures include:
  - Locked cabinets: Use secure cabinets to store implants, with access limited to authorised members of the surgical team.

- Dedicated storage areas: Separate implants so that they are not in direct contact with other items.

- Temperature and humidity control: Ensure that implants are stored in appropriate environmental conditions to prevent deterioration.

2. Labelling and traceability :
   - Each implant must be clearly labelled with essential information such as product name, batch number, expiry date and supplier. This facilitates traceability and rapid identification of implants.

3. Stock management systems :
   - Use computerised stock management systems to track implants electronically. These systems can monitor stock levels, manage replenishments and generate reports for efficient management.

4. Stock rotation :
   - Apply the "first in, first out" principle to ensure appropriate rotation of implants to minimise the risk of expiry.

5. Access control :
   - Restrict access to the implant storage area and monitor entry and exit activities using access control devices such as key card systems.

6. Staff training :
   - Train the surgical team in the correct identification, handling and documentation of implants. Also make staff aware of the importance of maintaining sterility when handling implants.

7. Usage reports :
   - Record every implant used in a surgical procedure, associating patient information with the specific implant used. This ensures complete and accurate traceability.

8. Monitoring product recalls :
   - Keep up to date with registered product recalls and ensure that the implants concerned are withdrawn from circulation and properly documented.

9. Data integration :
- Integrate implant information into patients' electronic medical records to ensure seamless communication between care teams.

Ensuring the safe storage and accurate traceability of implants is essential to guarantee patient safety, maintain the efficiency of surgical procedures and comply with regulatory standards. Proper management of implants contributes to the quality of care and the prevention of medical errors.

Accurate documentation of serial numbers and implant information is essential to ensure traceability, patient safety and regulatory compliance. Here's how to ensure rigorous documentation:

1. Initial registration :
- As soon as you receive the implants, record each implant in an electronic or manual tracking system. Collect information such as the manufacturer's name, batch number, date of manufacture, expiry date, product specifications and serial numbers.

2. Labelling :
- Each implant must be clearly labelled with all relevant information, including serial numbers. Use water- and wear-resistant labels to prevent information from fading.

3. Patient documentation :
- Link each implant to the patient's electronic medical record. Record the serial numbers associated with each surgical procedure, as well as the details of the operation.

4. Central database :
- Use a centralised database to record and store implant information. This database should be easily accessible to the authorised medical team.

5. Monitoring usage :
- Record the serial numbers of the implants used during each surgical procedure. Associate these numbers with patient records and surgical reports.

6. Updates :
   - Regularly update the database to reflect usage, inventory status and any product recalls.

7. Single numbering system :
   - Use a unique numbering system for implant serial numbers. This makes it easier to find and retrieve information.

8. Staff training :
   - Ensure that staff are trained to properly document implant information, including serial numbers, upon receipt and throughout the surgical process.

9. Reminder management :
   - Monitor product recalls and ensure that all affected implants are properly documented and withdrawn from use.

10. Systems integration :
   - If possible, integrate implant information into the hospital's existing electronic systems for optimum accessibility and communication.

Accurate documentation of implant serial numbers and information is an essential aspect of patient safety and surgical care management. Correct traceability means that implants can be identified quickly when needed, preventing errors and ensuring high-quality care.

Preparation of specific surgical equipment

Checking the anaesthesia, monitoring and suction devices is a crucial step before any surgical procedure begins, to ensure patient safety and the smooth running of the procedure. Here's how to do it:

1. Anaesthetic devices :
   - Check that the anaesthesia trolley is functional and correctly stocked with medicines, anaesthetic agents and essential equipment.

- Make sure that the anaesthesia circuit, face masks, balloons and tubes are clean, in good condition and ready for use.
- Check that the oxygen and anaesthetic delivery systems are working properly.
- Ensure that mechanical ventilation devices, such as the anaesthesia ventilator, are calibrated and ready for use.

2. Monitoring devices :
   - Check vital signs monitors such as heart rate, blood pressure, oxygen saturation and respiratory rate. Make sure they are switched on, working properly and calibrated.
   - Prepare the electrodes and sensors needed to monitor the patient's vital signs.
   - Check that the monitor alarms are correctly configured to warn of critical changes.

3. Suction devices :
   - Make sure that the suction devices are operational and that the drainage bottles are correctly installed.
   - Check that the cannulas and suction probes are ready for use and sterile.
   - Test the vacuum to ensure it is effective.

4. Documentation :
   - Document all checks carried out, including device serial numbers, functional checks and calibrations.

5. Staff training :
   - Make sure that the anaesthesia team is trained in the correct use of devices, the resolution of common problems and the management of emergency situations.

6. Communication :
   - Communicate clearly with the anaesthetic team and the surgical team about the condition and functionality of the devices.

7. Emergency stop procedure :
- Make sure that the anaesthetic team is familiar with the procedure for stopping anaesthetic devices in an emergency if necessary.

Careful checking of anaesthesia, monitoring and suction devices before surgery helps prevent technical problems during the procedure and ensures patient safety. It also enables the medical team to react quickly in the event of anomalies, malfunctions or emergency situations.

- Preparation of electrical instruments and cutting tools

Preparing electrical instruments and cutting tools in the operating theatre is a crucial step in ensuring patient safety and a successful surgical procedure. Here's how to do it effectively:

1. Initial inspection :
- Before the procedure, visually check the electrical instruments and cutting tools to make sure they are in good condition, clean and ready to use.

2. Correct operation :
- Test each electrical instrument to make sure it is working properly. Check the switches, speed settings and functions specific to each instrument.

3. Preventive maintenance :
- Make sure that electrical instruments have undergone regular preventive maintenance in accordance with the manufacturer's recommendations.

4. Cleaning and sterilisation :
- Before the procedure, make sure that the electrical instruments and cutting tools have been cleaned, disinfected and sterilised in accordance with asepsis protocols and sterilisation standards.

5. Preparation of the operating field :
- Prepare the operating field by placing the necessary electrical instruments and cutting tools within easy reach of the surgeon and the team.

6. Checking the electrical connection :
   - Make sure that the electrical instruments are correctly connected and that the power cables are in good condition.

7. Electrical safety :
   - Check that electrical sockets are in good condition and comply with safety standards. Use earthing devices to avoid electrical hazards.

8. Use in accordance with specifications :
   - Ensure that electrical instruments are used in accordance with the manufacturer's specifications and appropriate surgical practices.

9. Team informed :
   - Inform the surgical team of the specific details of the electrical instruments to be used, including their name, serial number and any special considerations.

10. Staff training :
    - Ensure that operating theatre staff are trained in the correct and safe use of electrical instruments, including handling techniques and safety precautions.

11. Documentation :
    - Document the preparation of electrical instruments and cutting tools in the patient's medical records and in the operating theatre registers.

Careful preparation of electrical instruments and cutting tools helps to minimise the risk of errors, ensure patient safety and optimise the surgical procedure.

Preventive maintenance and equipment troubleshooting

Planning regular maintenance of medical equipment in the operating theatre is essential to ensure that it works properly, prevents breakdowns and guarantees patient safety. Here's how to draw up an effective maintenance plan:

1. Equipment inventory :
   - Draw up a complete list of medical equipment in the operating theatre, including instruments, anaesthetic devices, monitors, electrical equipment, etc.

2. Identifying maintenance requirements :
   - Identify the specific maintenance needs of each piece of equipment by referring to the manufacturer's recommendations, regulatory guidelines and industry standards.

3. Maintenance schedule :
   - Establish a regular maintenance schedule for each piece of equipment, determining the frequency of inspections, repairs and updates.

4. Preventive maintenance :
   - Incorporate planned preventive maintenance measures to avoid breakdowns. This can include cleaning, lubrication, calibration and replacement of worn parts.

5. Corrective maintenance :
   - Make provision for corrective maintenance in the event of breakdowns or malfunctions. Ensure that staff know how to report problems and who to contact.

6. Staff responsibilities :
   - Clearly define staff responsibilities with regard to equipment maintenance. Designate individuals or teams responsible for monitoring, carrying out and documenting maintenance.

7. Staff training :
   - Provide ongoing training for staff on equipment maintenance, focusing on good handling, maintenance and repair practices.

8. Monitoring and documentation :
   - Keep a detailed record of all maintenance activities, including dates, actions taken, parts replaced and problems solved.

9. Stop planning :
   - Plan the downtime needed to carry out more in-depth maintenance work without disrupting scheduled surgical procedures.

10. Quality control :
   - Establish quality control processes to check the effectiveness of the maintenance carried out and to ensure that the equipment is operating to the required standards.

11. Resources and suppliers :
   - Identify the necessary resources, including qualified maintenance suppliers and spare parts, to support the maintenance plan.

12. Periodic review :
   - Regularly review and adapt the maintenance plan in line with new information, best practice and manufacturer updates.

A well-developed maintenance plan ensures that medical equipment in the operating theatre operates reliably and safely, contributing to quality of care and patient safety.

Resolving equipment breakdowns during surgery is an essential skill for the surgical team, particularly operating theatre nurses. Here are the steps to follow to effectively manage equipment failure during a surgical procedure:

1. Keeping calm :
   - Stay calm and rational. A calm reaction will enable the team to resolve the situation more effectively.

2. Notify the team :
   - Immediately inform the surgeon, anaesthetist and other members of the surgical team of the equipment failure.

3. Ensuring patient safety :
   - If the equipment failure poses a risk to patient safety, take the necessary steps to ensure patient safety, such as stopping the procedure if appropriate.

4. Isolate the fault :
   - Identify the exact source of the fault by examining the equipment and checking connections, wires and components.

5. Workaround :
   - If possible, consider a workaround to maintain the stability of the procedure. For example, use other equipment or an alternative method if it is safe to do so.

6. Contact technical service :
   - If the fault cannot be resolved quickly, contact the appropriate technical service for assistance. Some equipment may require the intervention of a qualified technician.

7. Notify the surgical team:
   - Keep the surgical team informed of the situation and the measures taken to resolve the fault.

8. Draw up an emergency plan :
   - If the procedure cannot be continued due to the fault, ensure that an emergency plan is in place to stabilise the patient and complete the procedure if necessary.

9. Documentation :
   - Thoroughly document the fault, the actions taken to resolve it and the decisions taken to ensure patient safety.

10. Revaluation :
   - Once the fault has been rectified, check that the equipment is working properly before resuming the procedure.

11. Feedback :
   - After the surgery, discuss the equipment failure as a team, the measures taken and how it could be avoided in the future.

Effective management of equipment breakdowns requires rapid communication, sound decision-making and coordinated action by the surgical team. Patient safety is always the top priority.

Use of advanced medical technology

Training on state-of-the-art equipment such as robotics and advanced imaging in the operating theatre is essential to ensure the safe and effective use of these technologies. Here's how to plan and deliver the right training:

1. Identifying training needs :
   - Identify specific cutting-edge equipment used in the operating theatre, such as surgical robotics systems, advanced imaging equipment (scanner, MRI, etc.) and other emerging technologies.

2. Design of the training programme :
   - Develop a structured training programme that covers all aspects of equipment use, including handling, programming, calibration, safety protocols, etc.

3. Initial training :
   - Provide comprehensive initial training for members of the surgical team, including surgeons, nurses and technicians, to ensure a thorough understanding of equipment functionality and capabilities.

4. Practical training :
   - Include practical sessions to give participants hands-on experience of the equipment. Use simulators or training environments to reproduce realistic surgical scenarios.

5. Further training :
   - Make sure that training is ongoing, with regular updates to keep pace with technological developments, new features and best practice.

6. Group and individual sessions :
   - Organise group training sessions to cover the basics, as well as individual sessions to meet the specific needs of each participant.

7. Working with suppliers :
   - Work with equipment suppliers to obtain their expertise in designing the training programme and organising equipment-specific training sessions.

8. Documentation and teaching materials :
   - Provide reference documents, user manuals, troubleshooting guides and other educational resources to support training.

9. Skills assessment :
   - Regularly assess the skills acquired by participants, using practical tests or simulations to ensure they have mastered the equipment.

10. Encouraging experimentation :
   - Encourage participants to explore the functionality of the equipment in a safe and controlled way under supervision, which boosts their confidence and competence.

11. Feedback :
   - Encourage participants to share their experiences and questions with their peers, which promotes collective learning and the exchange of knowledge.

Training on state-of-the-art equipment requires an ongoing commitment to ensure that the surgical team is proficient in the use of these advanced technologies, helping to improve surgical outcomes and patient safety.

The integration of technology into surgical procedures has evolved considerably in recent years, leading to significant improvements in precision, efficiency and patient outcomes. Here's how technology is being integrated into surgical procedures:

1. Advanced imaging :
   - The use of advanced medical imaging such as computed tomography (CT), magnetic resonance imaging (MRI) and 3D images gives surgeons a detailed, real-time view of the working area, making it easier to plan and navigate during surgery.

2. Surgical robotics :
   - Surgical robotics systems help surgeons to perform surgical procedures with greater precision. These robots are controlled by surgeons using consoles, and enable finer, more stable movements.

3. Guidance and navigation :
 - Surgical guidance systems use visual or infrared cues to track the position of instruments and guide surgeons through the procedure.

4. Augmented and virtual reality :
 - Augmented and virtual reality technologies offer real-time 3D visualisations of the patient's anatomy, enabling surgeons to better understand the layout of internal structures.

5. Endoscopy and miniaturisation :
 - Miniaturised endoscopes and high-definition cameras provide clear, detailed internal images, reducing the need for major incisions.

6. Intra-operative imaging :
 - Intra-operative imaging devices allow surgeons to directly visualise the targeted area in real time, which is particularly useful in complex procedures.

7. Laser and energy :
 - Advanced laser and energy technologies are used to cut, coagulate or vaporise tissue during surgery, reducing bleeding and promoting faster recovery.

8. Robotic and remote-controlled instruments :
 - Robotic or remote-controlled instruments enable surgeons to perform precise, complex movements with great stability, even in confined spaces.

9. Telemedicine and remote collaboration :
 - Telemedicine technologies enable expert surgeons to guide and advise on procedures remotely, encouraging learning and collaboration.

10. Real-time data :
 - Sensors and monitors provide real-time vital data on the patient's vital signs, helping to make rapid, informed decisions.

11. Electronic documentation :
  • Electronic medical records and hospital information systems make it easier to manage information about patients, procedures and results.

The integration of technology into surgical procedures has transformed the way operations are carried out, enabling more precise, less invasive interventions with better outcomes for patients. However, it is crucial that members of the surgical team are trained in the use of these technologies to maximise their benefits and ensure their safe use.

Sustainable management of instruments and equipment

Extending the life of surgical instruments is essential to optimising their use and reducing the costs associated with their frequent replacement. Here are a few practical ways to achieve this:

1. Suitable handling and storage :
  • Handle instruments with care to avoid knocks and drops that could damage the sharp edges.

  • Store instruments in specific cases or suitable bins to protect them from dust, moisture and contaminants.

2. Regular maintenance and cleaning :
  • Clean instruments immediately after use in accordance with recommended procedures.

  • Use appropriate cleaning solutions and avoid corrosive or abrasive products.

  • Inspect the instruments for damage or wear after cleaning.

3. Correct sterilisation :
  • Follow the recommended sterilisation guidelines for each type of instrument.

  • Avoid excessively long sterilisation cycles which could damage the instruments.

4. Regular sharpening :
   - Make sure that sharp instruments are regularly sharpened to maintain their effectiveness and avoid more aggressive gestures that could damage them.

5. Appropriate use :
   - Use each instrument for its intended purpose. Avoid forcing an instrument to perform a task for which it is not designed.

6. Avoid prolonged immersion:
   - Avoid immersing instruments for long periods, as this can damage materials and mechanisms.

7. Lubrication and protection :
   - Use appropriate lubricants for articulated or mechanical instruments to reduce wear and facilitate movement.

   - Protect sharp instruments with caps or sleeves when not in use.

8. Regular inspection :
   - Implement regular inspection processes to identify damaged or worn instruments requiring repair or replacement.

9. Staff training :
   - Ensure that all operating theatre staff are trained in good practice for the use and care of instruments.

10. Documentation :
   - Keep a record of the life, use and maintenance of each instrument to help monitor their condition and make informed decisions.

By adopting these practices, surgical instruments can be kept in good condition, leading to more effective and safer operations. Paying particular attention to the maintenance and correct use of instruments will help to extend their life and ensure that they work at their best.

The management of medical waste has a significant environmental impact due to the potentially hazardous nature of the waste produced in healthcare establishments. Here's how medical waste management can have an impact on the environment:

1. Air, water and soil pollution :
   - Some medical waste, such as chemicals, expired or unused pharmaceuticals and disinfectants, can contaminate the air, water and soil when improperly disposed of.

2. Risks to human and animal health :
   - Improper disposal of medical waste can pose risks to human and animal health, as chemicals and pathogens can contaminate ecosystems and water sources.

3. Use of resources :
   - The management of medical waste requires resources such as water and energy for the treatment and disposal processes, which can contribute to the over-exploitation of natural resources.

4. Greenhouse gas emissions :
   - The processes involved in treating and incinerating medical waste can result in greenhouse gas emissions, contributing to climate change.

5. Improper disposal of needles and sharp objects :
   - Improper disposal of needles and other sharp objects can result in potentially fatal injuries to those involved in waste management, as well as to waste collectors.

6. Antibiotic resistance :
   - Medical waste containing drug residues, including antibiotics, can contribute to antibiotic resistance, a growing public health problem.

7. Impact on biodiversity :
   - The contamination of aquatic and terrestrial ecosystems by chemicals and medical waste can have an impact on biodiversity by altering habitats and endangering animal and plant species.

To reduce the environmental impact of medical waste management, it is crucial to implement safe, effective and environmentally sound waste management practices. This includes the appropriate sorting, collection, storage, treatment and disposal of medical waste, as well as promoting the responsible use of chemicals and medicines. Awareness and education of healthcare professionals, facility staff and the public are also essential to encourage environmentally sound medical waste management practices.

Monitoring and documentation of instruments and equipment

Using electronic tracking systems to manage surgical instruments can significantly improve efficiency, traceability and safety in the operating theatre. Here's how these systems can be used:

1. Identification and monitoring of instruments :
   • Each instrument can be fitted with an RFID (radio frequency identification) chip or a unique barcode, enabling its use, location and status to be tracked in real time.

2. Stock management :
   • Electronic systems can help manage stock levels in real time, automatically signalling when it's time to order new instruments.

3. Planning interventions :
   • Instruments required for a specific procedure can be identified and prepared in advance, avoiding unnecessary delays.

4. Loss and theft prevention :
   • Electronic systems can alert staff if an instrument leaves the operating theatre without authorisation, reducing the risk of loss or theft.

5. Maintenance and calibration follow-up :
   • The systems can record the dates on which instruments are serviced, sharpened or calibrated, guaranteeing that they work properly and safely.

6. Documentation and reports :
   - Information on instrument use can be automatically recorded and integrated into electronic medical records, facilitating the creation of reports and analyses.

7. Traceability and compliance :
   - Electronic tracking systems allow complete traceability of each instrument, which is crucial for compliance with safety and sterilisation standards.

8. Reminder management :
   - Electronic systems can automatically alert staff when an instrument is recalled for safety or quality reasons.

9. Reducing human error :
   - By automating the monitoring and management of instruments, the risks of human error, such as incorrect documentation or the use of non-sterile instruments, are reduced.

10. Improving efficiency :
   - Electronic systems provide rapid access to instrument information, reducing search time and helping to make more efficient use of resources.

The use of electronic tracking systems can contribute to better organisation, more accurate instrument management, increased safety and an overall improvement in processes within the operating theatre. However, it is essential to provide adequate training for staff to ensure correct and optimal use of these systems.

Keeping accurate records is essential to ensure traceability, compliance and safety in the operating theatre. Here's how to maintain effective records for these purposes:

1. Identification of instruments and equipment :
   - Each instrument and piece of equipment must be clearly identified with a serial number, barcode or RFID chip to enable accurate tracking.

2. Use of instruments :
   - Record details of each instrument use, including patient name, procedure type, date and time.

3. Sterilisation and disinfection :
   - Document the sterilisation and disinfection cycles for each instrument, indicating dates, methods used and results.

4. Maintenance and servicing :
   - Keep a record of instrument maintenance, sharpening and calibration operations, including dates and details.

5. Stock management :
   - Monitor instrument and equipment stock levels to avoid shortages and surpluses.

6. Compliance with standards :
   - Ensure that registers comply with current standards and regulations, particularly in terms of safety, sterilisation and waste management.

7. Patient traceability :
   - Associate each instrument used with a specific patient to enable full traceability in the event of problems or recalls.

8. Reports and analyses :
   - Use the logs to generate reports and analyses to identify trends, potential risks and areas for improvement.

9. Electronic integration :
   - If possible, use computerised systems to record information and automate the generation of reports.

10. Training and liability :
   - Ensure that all staff involved in the use, sterilisation and maintenance of instruments are properly trained and aware of the importance of keeping accurate records.

11. Shelf life :
   - Comply with the guidelines on how long records must be kept, ensuring that they are retained for as long as is necessary for traceability and compliance.

Accurate record keeping is crucial for patient safety, efficient resource management and compliance with standards and regulations. By following these practices, you contribute to a safer, more efficient and better organised operating theatre environment.

Chapter 8:
After surgery and post-operative care

Transitioning the patient to the recovery room

Preparing the patient for transfer to the recovery room is an important step in ensuring a smooth awakening and a safe transition after surgery. Here are the key stages in this preparation:

1. Continuous monitoring :
   - Before the transfer, make sure the patient's vital signs are stable and carefully monitor any changes in their state of health.

2. Checking the airways :
   - Make sure the patient's airway is clear and that they can breathe freely.

3. Extubation (if necessary) :
   - If the patient is intubated during surgery, prepare for extubation by following the appropriate protocols.

4. Pain management :
   - Administer pain medication as prescribed by your doctor, so that the patient is comfortable during the transfer.

5. Appropriate packaging :
   - Make sure the patient is dressed comfortably and correctly for the transfer, taking into account medical and safety considerations.

6. Documentation :
   - Accurately document the patient's condition, medicines administered, vital signs and any other relevant details in the medical record.

7. Preparing the equipment :
   - Gather all the equipment and documents needed for the transfer, including the patient's medical file, medicines, monitoring devices and oxygen equipment.

8. Communication :
   - Contact the recovery room team to inform them of the imminent transfer and share all relevant patient information.

9. Preparing the stretcher :
   - Make sure the stretcher is clean, comfortable and equipped with everything you need for the transfer, such as blankets and arm and leg supports.

10. Patient information :
   - Inform the patient about the transfer to the recovery room, reassure them about what is going to happen and answer any questions they may have.

11. Informed consent :
   - If necessary, obtain the informed consent of the patient or their legal representative for the transfer.

12. Transfer assistance :
   - If the patient is unable to move themselves, make sure you have enough staff to help them safely.

Once the patient is ready, transfer them with care and attention, following the facility's protocols. Seamless communication between the surgical team and the recovery room team is essential to ensure a smooth transition and continuity of care for the patient.

Communicating relevant information to the recovery team is crucial to ensuring the patient's safety and well-being during the post-operative phase. Here's how to communicate effectively with the recovery team:

1. Verbal report :
   - Before the patient is transferred to the recovery room, give a verbal report to the recovery nurse or anaesthetist. Provide essential information about the surgical procedure,

the patient's current condition, any medication administered, vital signs, potential problems and any other relevant information.

2. Medical file :
   * Ensure that the patient's medical file, including operating notes, prescriptions, test results and anaesthetic reports, is available and passed on to the recovery team.

3. Written reports :
   * If possible, draw up a written report or use standardised forms to pass on important information to the recovery team.

4. Patient identifiers :
   * Ensure that the patient's identity is clearly communicated, including full name, date of birth and any other unique identifiers.

5. Brief summary :
   * Give a brief summary of the operation, the duration of the procedure, any complications that arose during surgery and any particular problems encountered.

6. Drugs administered :
   * Inform the recovery team of the drugs administered during surgery, in particular analgesics, sedatives and anaesthetic agents.

7. Allergic reactions :
   * Report any known drug allergy or allergic reaction that occurred during surgery.

8. Fluids and losses :
   * Communicate details of fluids administered during surgery, as well as blood and fluid losses.

9. Monitoring and vital signs :
   * Share the latest vital signs recorded, including heart rate, blood pressure, oxygen saturation, temperature, etc.

10. Neurological condition :
   - Inform the recovery team of the patient's neurological state, particularly if there have been any changes in reflexes, consciousness or sensitivity.

11. Special procedures :
   - If any special procedures were carried out during surgery (for example, placement of a urinary catheter), make sure the recovery team is informed.

12. Specific considerations :
   - If the patient has special needs, dietary requirements, restrictions or other specific considerations, ensure that this information is shared.

Clear and concise communication of relevant information between the surgical team and the recovery team ensures a smooth transition and appropriate management of the patient during the post-operative phase.

Monitoring the patient's vital signs and condition

Regular monitoring of vital parameters is essential to ensure the safety and well-being of patients in the recovery room and throughout their post-operative recovery. Here's how to monitor vital signs effectively:

1. Heart rate (HR) :
   - Use a heart monitor to continuously monitor the patient's heart rate. A significant increase or abnormal decrease in heart rate may indicate cardiovascular problems or pain.

2. Blood pressure (BP) :
   - Measure your blood pressure at regular intervals using a blood pressure monitor. Significant variations in blood pressure may indicate haemodynamic instability.

3. Oxygen saturation (SaO2) :
   - Monitor the patient's oxygen saturation using a pulse oximeter. A drop in oxygen saturation may necessitate an increase in oxygen intake.

4. Respiratory rate (RR) :
  - Count the breaths per minute to assess the patient's respiratory rate. Abnormal changes may indicate breathing problems.

5. Body temperature :
  - Monitor your body temperature for signs of post-operative fever or hypothermia.

6. Level of awareness :
  - Regularly assess the patient's level of consciousness by observing their reactivity, state of alertness and ability to respond to stimuli.

7. Pain :
  - Ask the patient to report their pain level using a standard pain scale. Adjust analgesics accordingly.

8. Airways :
  - Monitor the patient's breathing and make sure the airway remains clear to prevent any breathing problems.

9. Volume of urine :
  - Record urine volume to assess renal function and hydration.

10. Allergic or adverse reactions :
  - Be alert for signs of allergic or adverse reactions to drugs administered during surgery.

11. Response to stimuli :
  - Regularly check the patient's response to stimuli, assessing their ability to move, respond verbally and open their eyes.

12. Precise documentation :
  - Accurately record all measurements in the patient's medical record, including times of readings and specific observations.

13. Appropriate answers :
  - In the event of abnormalities or significant fluctuations in vital parameters, immediately inform the doctor or medical team for rapid assessment and intervention.

Regular, careful monitoring of vital parameters means that any changes in the patient's condition can be detected quickly and prompt action taken to prevent or treat post-operative complications. This plays a crucial role in the overall management of the patient during the recovery period.

Assessing the patient's pain and reaction to anaesthesia is an important step in ensuring their comfort and safety during the post-operative phase. Here's how to do it:

1. Early assessment :
   - As soon as the patient is transferred to the recovery room, begin with an initial assessment of their pain and level of consciousness.

2. Using a pain scale :
   - Ask the patient to rate their pain on a scale of 0 to 10, where 0 represents no pain and 10 represents the worst pain imaginable. This can give you an indication of the severity of the pain experienced.

3. Observation of signs of pain :
   - Look for non-verbal signs of pain, such as grimacing, muscle tension, rapid or shallow breathing and restless movements.

4. Verbal communication :
   - Encourage patients to express their pain verbally and ask them to describe the nature, location and intensity of their pain.

5. Assessment of response to anaesthesia :
   - Observe the patient's reactions to the anaesthetic, such as their level of consciousness, breathing and oxygen saturation. Make sure the patient wakes up gently and safely.

6. Communication with the anaesthetist :
   - If complications related to anaesthesia are observed (e.g. breathing difficulties, allergic reactions), contact the anaesthetist immediately for advice and instructions.

7. Administration of analgesics :
  - If the patient reports pain, administer the prescribed analgesics in accordance with medical prescriptions.

8. Frequent reassessment :
  - Reassess the patient's pain regularly after administering analgesics to check their effectiveness and adjust the dosage if necessary.

9. Continuous observation :
  - Monitor the patient's vital signs constantly during this critical period, paying particular attention to breathing, oxygen saturation and blood pressure.

10. Emotional support :
  - Provide the patient with emotional support and reassuring explanations of their situation, answering their questions and helping them to manage their worries.

Assessing the patient's pain and response to anaesthesia requires careful communication and continuous monitoring to ensure that the patient wakes up comfortably and safely after surgery.

Post-operative pain management

Administering and monitoring analgesics in accordance with protocols is essential to effectively manage patients' post-operative pain and ensure their comfort. Here are the key steps to administering and monitoring analgesics appropriately:

1. Medical prescription :
  - Before administering any analgesic, make sure you have a precise, up-to-date medical prescription indicating the type of analgesic, the dose, the route of administration and the frequency.

2. Choice of analgesic :
  - Select the appropriate analgesic according to the severity of the pain, the patient's medical history and any known allergies.

3. Route of administration :
- Analgesics can be administered orally, intravenously, intramuscularly, subcutaneously or epidurally, depending on the protocols and the patient's needs.

4. Patient education :
- Inform the patient about the type of analgesic being administered, its mode of action, possible side effects and the steps to be taken to report any adverse reactions.

5. Precise administration :
- Strictly adhere to the prescribed dosage and the time intervals between doses. Use appropriate measuring devices to ensure accurate administration.

6. Continuous monitoring :
- Monitor the patient's vital signs regularly, in particular heart rate, blood pressure, oxygen saturation and respiration, after each administration of analgesic.

7. Pain assessment :
- Ask patients regularly about their pain levels and how they feel after the analgesic has been administered. Use pain scales to quantify and monitor pain intensity.

8. Revaluation and adjustment :
- Depending on the patient's response to the analgesic, adjust the dosage if necessary to improve pain control while minimising side effects.

9. Prevention of side effects :
- Watch out for potential side effects such as sedation, nausea, vomiting, itching and dizziness and act accordingly.

10. Precise documentation :
- Systematically record the times and doses administered, the patient's responses, the interventions taken and any side-effects observed in the patient's medical record.

11. Interdisciplinary communication :
- Communicate with the medical team, including doctors, nurses and pharmacists, to discuss the effectiveness of pain management and adjust treatment plans if necessary.

The administration and monitoring of analgesics must be carried out diligently and carefully to ensure adequate pain relief, minimise the risk of side effects and promote the patient's comfortable recovery from surgery.

In addition to analgesics, there are a number of non-pharmacological techniques that are effective in reducing post-operative pain and improving patient comfort. These techniques can be used alone or in combination with medication, depending on the patient's needs and preferences. Here are some of these non-pharmacological techniques:

1. Relaxation and deep breathing :
   - Teach the patient progressive muscle relaxation and deep breathing techniques to reduce anxiety and muscle tension, which can help to reduce pain.

2. Distraction techniques :
   - Suggest distracting activities such as reading, listening to soothing music, watching videos or playing mental games to divert the patient's attention from the pain.

3. Guided imagery :
   - Guide the patient in using the imagination to create positive and relaxing mental images, which can help reduce the perception of pain.

4. Massage therapy :
   - Use gentle massage techniques to relax muscles and stimulate the release of endorphins, the body's natural painkillers.

5. Acupuncture and acupressure :
   - Apply pressure or use needles on specific points on the body to stimulate energy flow and relieve pain.

6. TENS (Transcutaneous Electrical Nerve Stimulation) :
   - Use electrodes to send weak electrical currents through the skin, which can help block pain signals.

7. Heat and cold :
   - Apply hot or cold compresses to the painful area to relieve pain and reduce inflammation.

8. Yoga and meditation :
   - Teach the patient gentle yoga exercises and meditation techniques to promote relaxation and self-awareness, which can help reduce pain.

9. Hypnosis :
   - Guide the patient into an altered state of consciousness to encourage deep relaxation and reduce the perception of pain.

10. Massage therapy :
   - Provide professional massages to relax muscles and stimulate blood circulation, which can reduce pain.

It is important to discuss with the patient and work closely with the medical team to select appropriate non-pharmacological techniques based on the patient's condition, the nature of the surgery and personal preferences. These complementary approaches can play a significant role in managing post-operative pain and improving the patient's overall well-being.

Care of incisions and dressings

Inspecting and cleaning surgical incisions is an integral part of post-operative care to prevent infection and promote optimal healing. Here are the steps to follow to properly inspect and clean surgical incisions:

1. Preparation :
   - Before you start, make sure your hands are clean by washing thoroughly with soap and water or using a hand sanitiser.

2. Setting up a clean environment :
   - Choose a clean, well-lit area for inspection and cleaning. Use sterile gloves and wear a mask if necessary.

3. Visual inspection :
   - Carefully examine the incision for signs of infection, inflammation, dehiscence (opening of the incision) or abnormal drainage. Look for redness, swelling, excessive heat or the presence of pus.

4. Cleaning the incision :
   - If the incision needs cleaning, use a mild antiseptic solution recommended by your healthcare professional. Soak a sterile compress in the solution and gently clean around the incision, avoiding excessive rubbing.

5. Use of asepsis :
   - Handle the incision with care to avoid contamination. Use a clean compress for each pass to avoid spreading germs.

6. Drying :
   - Leave the incision to air-dry or gently pat dry with a clean sterile compress. Do not rub the area.

7. Application of a sterile dressing :
   - If necessary, apply a sterile dressing recommended by the healthcare professional to protect the incision. Make sure it fits snugly and is not too tight.

8. Documentation :
   - Take precise notes on the state of the incision, any unusual observations and the measures taken. This information should be recorded in the patient's medical record.

9. Continuous monitoring :
   - Monitor the incision regularly for any changes in its appearance or condition. Report any signs of infection or complications to the medical team immediately.

10. Patient education :
   - Instruct the patient on the signs of infection to look out for at home, how to clean the incision if necessary, and how often to report to the medical team.

Inspecting and cleaning surgical incisions are crucial steps in maintaining patient health and preventing complications. Be sure to follow the protocols recommended by the medical team and communicate any concerns or changes observed in the incision.

Applying sterile dressings and monitoring healing are essential steps in ensuring optimal healing of surgical incisions. Here are the steps to follow to apply sterile dressings and monitor healing appropriately:

1. Preparation :
   • Before you start, make sure your hands are clean by washing thoroughly with soap and water or using a hand sanitiser.

2. Setting up a clean environment :
   • Choose a clean, well-lit area to apply the dressing. Use sterile gloves and wear a mask if necessary.

3. Removing the old dressing :
   • If a previous dressing is in place, remove it carefully, avoiding any sudden movements that could damage the scar or cause pain.

4. Cleaning the area :
   • Gently clean the area around the scar with a mild antiseptic solution recommended by the healthcare professional. Use a sterile compress to avoid contamination.

5. Drying :
   • Leave the area to air dry or gently pat dry with a clean sterile compress. Do not rub the scar.

6. Applying the sterile dressing :
   • Apply a sterile dressing recommended by the medical team to the scar. Make sure it fits snugly and covers the area completely.

7. Healing follow-up :
   • Check the scar regularly for signs of infection, dehiscence or healing problems. Look for redness, swelling, abnormal fluid secretion or pus discharge.

8. Documentation :
   • Take precise notes on the condition of the scar, any unusual observations and the measures taken. This information should be recorded in the patient's medical file.

9. Patient education :
  - Instruct the patient on how to care for the scar at home, what signs of infection to look out for and how often to report to the medical team.

10. Dressing change :
  - Follow the medical team's instructions on how and how often to change the dressing. Make sure you maintain strict hygiene when changing the dressing.

11. Promoting healing :
  - Encourage the patient to maintain a balanced diet, stay hydrated and avoid smoking, which can promote optimal healing.

12. Medical consultation :
  - If any scarring problems are detected, contact the medical team immediately for further advice and care.
  -

The application of sterile dressings and careful monitoring of healing are essential to avoid complications and promote successful recovery. Working closely with the medical team and following recommended protocols will ensure effective management of post-operative healing.

Prevention of post-surgical complications

To avoid infections, blood clots and other post-operative complications, a number of preventive measures need to be put in place. Here are some important strategies for minimising risks and promoting a smooth recovery for patients:

Infection prevention :
  - **Hand hygiene:** Practice strict hand hygiene using soap and water or a hand disinfectant before and after any contact with the patient or instruments.

  - **Asepsis:** Strictly observe asepsis protocols when preparing and handling instruments and applying dressings to avoid contamination.

- **Prophylactic antibiotics:** Administer prophylactic antibiotics in accordance with medical guidelines prior to surgery to prevent infection.

- **Environmental control:** Make sure the operating theatre is clean and sterile. Control temperature, humidity and air filtration to reduce the risk of infection.

- **Appropriate use of equipment :** Check that all equipment is clean, sterile and working properly. Avoid contaminated or poorly maintained equipment.

Prevention of blood clots (deep vein thrombosis - DVT) :
- **Early mobility:** Encourage patients to move and walk as soon as possible after surgery to prevent clots from forming.

- **Support stockings:** Use support stockings to improve blood circulation and reduce the risk of blood clots.

- **Thromboprophylaxis:** Administer prophylactic anticoagulant medication according to medical guidelines to reduce the risk of blood clots.

- **Exercise:** Teach patients simple exercises, such as ankle-bending movements, to stimulate blood circulation when they are bedridden.

Prevention of other complications :
- **Medical monitoring:** Carry out regular medical check-ups to monitor the patient's condition and detect any complications at an early stage.

- **Pressure sore prevention:** Regularly change the patient's position and use special mattresses to prevent pressure sores.

- **Pain management:** Make sure the patient receives adequate pain management to avoid pain-related complications such as respiratory retention.

- **Preventing pneumonia:** Encourage deep breathing and coughing exercises to prevent postoperative pneumonia.

- **Hydration:** Maintain adequate hydration to promote blood circulation and healing.

- **Patient education:** Instruct patients on the signs of complications to look out for and the steps to take in the event of a problem.

- **Prevention of confusion:** For elderly patients, put in place measures to prevent confusion and delirium after the operation.

It is essential that the medical team works closely together to implement these preventive measures. As each patient is unique, protocols may vary depending on the patient's state of health, the type of surgery and other individual factors. By rigorously following these measures, it is possible to significantly reduce the risk of post-operative complications.

Early mobilisation and breathing exercises are essential measures for reducing the risk of complications after surgery. They promote blood circulation, prevent infections, reduce the risk of blood clots and improve lung function. Here's how to use them effectively:

Early mobilisation :
- **Early assessment:** As soon as the patient is medically stable, assess their ability to move and stand. Identify the patient's specific needs according to their state of health and the nature of the surgery.

- **Mobilisation plan:** Draw up a personalised mobilisation plan for each patient, taking into account their effort tolerance and physical strength. Encourage progressive mobilisation, starting with simple movements.

- **Mobilisation assistance:** If necessary, provide assistance to help the patient get up, sit at the edge of the bed and walk, using assistive devices if required.

- **Frequency:** Encourage patients to get up and walk around several times a day. Regular movement promotes blood circulation and prevents stagnation.

- **Preventing falls:** Ensure patient safety by providing appropriate assistance and using devices such as grab rails.

Breathing exercises :
- **Deep breathing exercises:** Teach the patient deep breathing exercises to prevent pulmonary complications. The exercises consist of breathing in slowly through the nose, holding the air for a few seconds and then breathing out slowly through the mouth.

- **Assisted cough:** Show the patient how to cough effectively to clear secretions and prevent pneumonia. Encourage them to use an assisted coughing technique, placing their hands on their abdomen to help expel secretions.

- **Deep breathing exercises in position:** Encourage the patient to perform deep breathing exercises while changing position (sitting, standing) to strengthen the respiratory muscles.

- **Incentive spirometry:** Use an incentive spirometer to help patients visualise their lung capacity and monitor progress.

- **Ongoing education:** Make sure the patient understands the importance of breathing exercises and encourage regular practice, even after discharge from hospital.

Early mobilisation and breathing exercises must be adapted to the patient's condition and the nature of the surgery. They are an integral part of post-operative management to reduce complications and speed up the recovery process. The medical team, including operating theatre nurses, plays an essential role in encouraging and supervising these beneficial practices.

Managing the side effects of anaesthesia

Monitoring and treating nausea, vomiting and other adverse events after surgery is crucial for the patient's well-being and to prevent complications. Post-operative nausea and vomiting

(PONV) are common reactions to anaesthesia and surgery. Here's how to monitor and treat them effectively:

Monitoring :
- **Early assessment:** As soon as the patient starts to wake up from anaesthesia, watch carefully for signs of nausea, vomiting or malaise.

- **Risk factors:** Identify risk factors that increase the likelihood of PONV, such as a history of previous postoperative nausea, major abdominal surgery, duration of surgery and type of anaesthetic used.

- **Communication with the patient:** Inform the patient that nausea and vomiting may occur after surgery. Encourage them to report any symptoms as soon as they occur.

- **Ongoing assessment:** Continuously monitor the patient's vital signs and observe any changes in their condition, including verbal or non-verbal signs of discomfort.

Treatment :
- **Prevention:** If the patient has high risk factors, consider administering prophylactic anti-nausea medication before or during surgery, in accordance with medical protocols.

- **Administration of medication: In the** event of nausea or vomiting, administer anti-nausea medication according to medical guidelines. These may include serotonin receptor antagonists, dopamine receptor antagonists or other agents.

- **Hydration:** Make sure the patient remains adequately hydrated. Intravenous fluids can help prevent dehydration due to vomiting.

- **Light food:** Offer the patient light, non-irritating food once symptoms have subsided. Avoid fatty or spicy foods that could aggravate nausea.
- **Repositioning:** Help the patient get into a more comfortable position, for example by raising the head of the bed, to relieve nausea.

- **Distraction:** Offer distraction techniques, such as soft music or visualisation, to help reduce anxiety and nausea.

- **Ongoing monitoring:** After administering anti-nausea medication, monitor the effectiveness of the treatment and react accordingly. Make sure the patient is comfortable and well hydrated.

- **Education:** Instruct the patient on self-care measures to reduce the risk of nausea and vomiting, including slow movement, hydration and eating light meals.

As an operating theatre nurse, your role is essential in monitoring and managing symptoms of nausea, vomiting and other post-operative side effects. Communication with the medical team and patient education are key to ensuring a smooth recovery and minimising complications related to these symptoms.

Comforting the patient and providing reassuring information are crucial aspects of the operating theatre nurse's role. Patients can be anxious and uncertain before surgery, and your compassionate presence can have a significant impact on their experience. Here's how you can do this effectively:

Before surgery :
- **Establish a connection:** Take the time to talk to the patient and create a bond of trust. Listen carefully to their concerns and answer their questions.

- **Pre-operative education:** Explain the stages of the surgical procedure, the sensations he might feel under anaesthetic, the measures taken to ensure his safety, and the presence of the competent medical team.

- **Active listening:** Be attentive to the patient's concerns and encourage them to express their emotions. Listen without judgement and offer empathetic support.

- **Detailed information:** Provide precise information on preparations before surgery, post-operative care and measures taken to minimise pain and complications.

In the operating theatre :
- **Reassuring presence:** Be by the patient's side as they prepare for surgery, holding their hand if necessary. Reassure them about the procedure.

- **Soothing communication:** Use a calm and reassuring tone of voice to talk to the patient while they are under anaesthetic. Explain that the team is there to look after him.

- **Accompanying the anaesthetic:** If the patient is conscious when the anaesthetic is administered, stay by their side to reassure them. Explain the process and encourage them to concentrate on their breathing.

After surgery :
- **Gentle awakening:** Once the surgery is over, be present when the patient regains consciousness. Explain briefly that the procedure is over and that everything went well.

- **Physical comfort:** Use gentle gestures to comfort the patient, such as adjusting their pillow or helping them to position themselves comfortably.

- **Empathetic communication:** As soon as the patient is awake, start a gentle, reassuring conversation. Inform them of the results of the surgery if appropriate.
- **Pain prevention:** Explain the measures taken to manage post-operative pain and reassure patients that their comfort is a priority.

- **Availability:** Make sure the patient knows that they can call you if they need to and that you are there to answer their questions and concerns.

Your role as an operating theatre nurse goes beyond the technical aspects. Providing emotional support and reassuring information creates an environment conducive to patient confidence and recovery. Your compassion and comforting presence can make a significant contribution to improving the overall patient experience.

Patient and family education

After surgery, post-operative care plays a crucial role in the patient's recovery. As an operating theatre nurse, you play a vital role in providing information about care, medication and restrictions. Here are a few things to bear in mind:

Post-operative care :
- **Continuous monitoring:** Explain to the patient that he or she will be monitored in the recovery room and in the post-anaesthesia unit to ensure that his or her condition is stabilised.

- **Positioning:** Give instructions on the best position for resting, depending on the surgery performed. Encourage regular changes of position to prevent complications.

- **Nutrition and hydration:** Explain the instructions for post-operative nutrition and hydration. In some cases, the patient may be allowed to drink clear liquids before gradually switching to a solid diet.

- **Deep breathing and coughing:** Encourage deep breathing and coughing exercises to prevent lung complications and help eliminate secretions.

Medicines :
- **Analgesics:** Explain to the patient the drugs prescribed to relieve post-operative pain. Give instructions on the frequency and dose to be taken, as well as on how to manage any side effects.

- **Antibiotics:** If antibiotics are prescribed, inform the patient of the importance of following the full dosage regimen to prevent infection.

- **Anticoagulants:** For patients at risk of blood clots, explain the use of anticoagulants, the warning signs of excessive bleeding and the steps to take.

Restrictions and precautions :
- **Physical activity:** Give clear guidelines on restrictions to physical activity, particularly with regard to lifting heavy objects and sudden movements.

- **Personal hygiene:** Explain how to take showers or baths without getting incisions or dressings wet.

- **Avoiding infection:** Give advice on how to care for surgical incisions, avoid exposure to stagnant water and identify signs of potential infection.

- **Medical follow-up:** Inform the patient about follow-up appointments with the doctor and the need to report any changes or complications.

- **Diet and medication:** If dietary restrictions or drug interactions are necessary, clearly explain these guidelines.

- **Emergency signs:** Educate the patient about symptoms that require immediate medical attention, such as excessive bleeding, high fever or severe pain.

Effective communication of this information is essential to ensure the patient's safe recovery from surgery. By providing clear instructions, answering the patient's questions and offering ongoing support, you are helping to ensure the patient's well-being during this critical period.

Preparing patients and their families for the transition home after surgery is an essential step in ensuring a successful recovery. As an operating theatre nurse, you play a crucial role in this process. Here's how you can help prepare the patient and family for this transition:

- **Early education:** As soon as the patient is conscious after surgery, start providing information about home care and the measures to be taken to facilitate optimum recovery.

- **Incision care:** Give detailed instructions on how to care for surgical incisions, including how to clean, change dressings and monitor for signs of infection.

- **Medication:** Review the medicines prescribed and explain how to take them correctly, including doses, times and any side effects to watch out for.

- **Physical activities:** Give guidelines on the physical activities permitted and the restrictions to be followed. Explain the importance of balancing rest and mobility.

- **Nutrition and hydration:** Provide advice on the types of food to eat, adequate hydration and any dietary restrictions.

- **Pain and comfort:** Discuss measures for managing pain at home, including prescribed analgesics and non-pharmacological techniques.

- **Warning signs:** Inform the patient and family of signs that require immediate medical attention, such as excessive bleeding, signs of infection or respiratory complications.

- **Medical follow-up:** Schedule follow-up appointments with the doctor and make sure the patient and family understand the importance of these visits to monitor healing and adjust care if necessary.

- **Home help:** If the patient requires home help or ongoing care, provide information on the options available and help coordinate the necessary arrangements.

- **Emotional support:** Offer emotional support to the patient and their family, and encourage them to express their concerns and needs.

- **Coordination with follow-up care:** Ensure that all relevant information is passed on to the healthcare professionals who will continue to monitor the patient.

- **Documentation:** Provide written instructions so that the patient can refer to the information at home. Make sure the patient has all the necessary contacts in case of questions or concerns.

Preparing the patient and family for the transition home is an important step in ensuring a safe recovery and continuity of care. Your role as an operating theatre nurse in this process is to provide clear information, emotional support and coordinate the care needed to ensure the patient's well-being once they leave hospital.

Transfer of the patient to the care unit

Preparing the patient for transfer out of the recovery room is a crucial step in ensuring a safe recovery. As an operating theatre nurse, here's how you can help:

- **Patient stability:** Before transfer, ensure that the patient is haemodynamically, respiratorily and neurologically stable. All vital parameters must be monitored and within acceptable ranges.

- **Post-anaesthetic assessment:** Check that the patient has recovered sufficiently from anaesthesia to allow safe transfer. Ensure that transfer criteria are met.

- **Equipment preparation:** Ensure that the patient is properly equipped for the transfer, including continuous monitoring devices such as cardiac, oxygen saturation and blood pressure monitors.

- **Information for staff:** Provide a detailed report to the post-anaesthesia care unit staff on the patient's current condition, the medication administered, the procedures performed and the patient's responses.

- **Wake-up stimulation:** If necessary, encourage the patient to slowly regain consciousness, open their eyes and respond verbally before the transfer.

- **Emotional support:** Make sure the patient feels safe and comfortable before the transfer. Briefly explain the transfer procedure and answer any questions.

- **Airway check: Make** sure the patient's airway is clear and breathing is stable.

- **Haemodynamic stability:** If the patient has received fluids or medication to maintain blood pressure, ensure that blood pressure is stable and that there are no signs of excessive bleeding.

- **Comfort:** Make sure the patient is comfortably installed on a stretcher or transfer bed, with cushions to support the necessary parts of the body.

- **Coordination:** Work with the post-anaesthesia care team to ensure a smooth and seamless transfer. Make sure all the necessary equipment is ready for transfer.

- **Written report:** Provide a detailed written report on the patient's current condition, the procedures carried out, the medication administered and the patient's responses. Ensure that all essential information is communicated.

- **Instructions for the patient:** If possible, give the patient instructions on what to expect when they arrive in the post-anaesthetic care unit and how they can participate in their recovery.

Preparing the patient for transfer out of the recovery room requires effective communication, careful assessment and coordination between members of the care team. Your role is to ensure that the patient is physically and emotionally ready for this important transfer to the next phase of their recovery.

Passing on crucial information to the post-anaesthetic care unit team is an essential step in ensuring continuity of care and the patient's safe recovery. As an operating theatre nurse, here's how you can pass on this information effectively:

- **Verbal report:** Before the patient is transferred, provide a detailed verbal report to the nurse in the post-anaesthetic care unit. Talk about the patient's current condition, the medication administered, the anaesthetic received, the patient's responses and any events or complications that occurred during the surgery.
- **Written documentation:** Prepare a full written report in the patient's medical file. Include details of procedures,

223

drugs, dosages, patient responses, equipment used, any complications and any other relevant information.

- **Vital parameters:** Transmit the patient's latest vital parameters, including heart rate, blood pressure, oxygen saturation and respiratory rate.

- **Medical history:** Inform the post-anaesthesia care team of the patient's medical history, including allergies, pre-existing illnesses, current medication and any medical conditions that may affect post-operative care.

- **Laboratory tests:** If laboratory tests have been carried out, please provide the relevant results, such as haemoglobin levels, electrolytes, blood gases, etc.

- **Fluids and medication:** Provide information on intravenous fluids administered, medications and doses given during surgery.

- **Specific equipment:** If specific equipment was used during surgery, such as drains or monitoring devices, make sure that the post-anaesthesia care unit team is aware of this and knows how to manage it.

- **Care plan:** Briefly explain the post-operative care plan, including analgesic requirements, permitted activities, restrictions and next steps in recovery.

- **Patient reactions:** Inform the team of any unusual reactions or changes in the patient's condition during surgery or during recovery.
- **Questions and concerns:** Make sure the post-anaesthesia care unit team knows where to contact you if you have any questions or concerns.

- **Coordination:** Working closely with the nurse in the post-anaesthesia care unit to facilitate a smooth transfer and ensure fluid communication.

- **Empathy and support:** Show empathy towards the patient and the post-anaesthesia care unit team and make sure that the team feels supported in the care of the patient.

Accurate and complete transmission of crucial information ensures that the post-anaesthesia care unit team has all the information it needs to provide high-quality patient care during the recovery phase and beyond. Your effective communication contributes to consistent and safe care throughout the patient journey.

Post-operative follow-up and follow-up appointments

Planning follow-up consultations with doctors and specialists is an important step in ensuring the patient's continued and full recovery after surgery. As an operating theatre nurse, you can contribute to this process in the following ways:

- **Early coordination:** As soon as the date for surgery has been set, start coordinating with the doctors and specialists involved in post-operative care. Identify the patient's specific needs in terms of medical follow-up.

- **Communication with doctors:** Contact the doctors responsible for monitoring the patient to discuss the operation, results, post-operative recommendations and any specialist consultation needs.

- **Appointment scheduling:** Help plan follow-up appointments with doctors and specialists, taking into account medical requirements and patient availability.

- **Preparing information:** Prepare a complete patient medical record, including test results, surgical reports, prescribed medication and any other relevant information, to share with follow-up doctors.

- **Passing on information:** Provide the follow-up doctors with all the necessary information on the surgery, potential complications, procedures carried out and medicines administered.

- **Interdisciplinary cooperation:** Work closely with the nurses in the post-anaesthesia care unit and the care team in the surgical unit to ensure a smooth transition to medical follow-up.

- **Follow-up appointments:** Make sure that patients are informed of their follow-up appointments and that they have all the necessary information, including doctors' contact details and appointment details.

- **Coordination of results:** When the results of follow-up consultations are available, ensure that they are properly documented in the patient's medical record and shared with the relevant members of the medical team.

- **Answering questions:** Answer the patient's questions about follow-up appointments, medical recommendations and post-operative care.
- **Patient education:** Inform the patient about the importance of follow-up consultations, the objectives of each consultation and the benefits of regular medical monitoring.

- **Ongoing monitoring:** Keep in touch with the patient after surgery to ensure that he or she is following medical recommendations and carrying out follow-up consultations as planned.

- **Two-way communication:** Make sure that doctors and specialists also communicate with you about the results of follow-up consultations and additional recommendations.

Effective planning and coordination of follow-up consultations is essential to ensure that the patient receives appropriate medical care after surgery. Your role in communication, documentation and coordination contributes to a smooth transition to post-operative care and to the overall success of the patient's recovery.

Monitoring patient progress and resolving concerns are crucial aspects of your role as an operating theatre nurse. Here's how you can do this effectively:

- **Regular communication:** Maintain regular communication with the patient and those around them to monitor progress and resolve concerns. Listen carefully to their feedback and questions.

- **Careful observation:** Monitor vital signs, pain levels, reactions to medication and any other changes in the patient's condition during the post-operative period.

- **Accurate documentation:** Carefully document all details of the patient's condition, the care provided, the medicines administered and the patient's responses in the medical record.

- **Systematic assessment:** Carry out regular assessments of the patient's condition in accordance with established protocols, noting improvements, challenges and concerns.

- **Responding to concerns:** When the patient or family expresses concerns, listen carefully, clarify the points of concern and ensure that appropriate action is taken to resolve them.

- **Communication with the medical team:** Communicate with doctors and other members of the medical team to discuss the patient's concerns and develop an appropriate action plan.

- **Ongoing education:** Provide ongoing information to the patient and family about the stages of recovery, permitted activities, care at home, signs of complications and precautions to be taken.

- **Referrals required:** If specific medical needs arise, ensure that the patient is referred to the appropriate specialists for a thorough assessment.

- **Empathy and support:** Show empathy towards the patient and their family, offer emotional support and respond to their needs for information and care.

- **Interdisciplinary collaboration:** Work closely with the nurses in the post-anaesthesia care unit and other members of the care team to ensure comprehensive, coordinated patient care.

- **Long-term follow-up:** Monitoring the patient's progress can continue after discharge from hospital. Make sure you provide clear instructions for home care and schedule follow-up appointments if necessary.

- **Overall assessment:** As the patient recovers, assess their overall condition, physical and psychological well-being, and ensure that they are achieving their recovery goals.

As an operating theatre nurse, your role doesn't end with the end of surgery. Carefully monitoring the patient's progress and resolving concerns quickly contributes significantly to a smooth recovery and patient satisfaction. Your ongoing involvement and attentive care play an essential role in the healing process.

Chapter 9:
Professional development and ethics

Commitment to continuing education

Keeping up to date with medical advances and new practices is essential for operating theatre nurses. This ensures the delivery of high quality care, patient safety and effective professional practice. Here's why it's so important:

- **Patient safety:** Medical advances are leading to better surgical techniques, more effective medicines and improved safety protocols, reducing the risks to patients.

- **Best practices:** New practices are often based on current scientific evidence, which means that you are using the most effective methods to deliver patient care.

- **Reducing errors:** By keeping abreast of new methods and technologies, you can avoid potential medical errors and implement appropriate preventive measures.

- **Optimised care:** Access to the latest information enables you to optimise care, reduce intervention time and promote faster patient recovery.

- **Adapting to new technologies:** Medical advances often include the use of cutting-edge technologies. Being informed helps you to familiarise yourself with these tools and to use them competently.

- **Evolving standards:** Protocols and standards of care evolve over time. Keeping up to date allows you to comply with current standards and ensure ethical practice.

- **Continuous improvement:** By incorporating new knowledge into your practice, you promote continuous improvement in your skills and the quality of your care.

- **Professional leadership:** By being at the cutting edge of medical advances, you can share your knowledge with your peers, becoming a leader in your field.

- **Patient confidence:** Patients tend to have more confidence in informed and up-to-date healthcare professionals.

- **Professional development:** Constantly seeking out new knowledge and skills contributes to your own professional development and job satisfaction.

- **Responses to challenges:** Medicine is constantly evolving, and being up to date prepares you to face new challenges and make informed decisions.

- **Professional ethics:** By staying informed, you meet your ethical obligation to provide care based on the best available evidence.

To stay up to date, take part in regular continuing education courses, attend conferences, read medical journals, follow new guidelines and collaborate with your colleagues to exchange knowledge. Your commitment to staying informed makes a significant contribution to improving patient care and advancing the profession of operating theatre nursing.

Attending conferences, workshops and training programmes is essential for operating theatre nurses. It enables them to keep up to date with the latest medical advances, improve their skills and enhance their professional practice. Here's how these activities can benefit OR nurses:

- **Updating your knowledge:** Conferences, workshops and training programmes keep you abreast of new research, medical discoveries and best practices, so you can keep your knowledge up to **date.**

- **Continuous learning:** These events offer continuous learning opportunities, helping you to acquire new skills and improve your professional practice.

- **New techniques:** Practical workshops give you the opportunity to learn new surgical techniques, improve your instrument skills and discover innovative approaches.

- **Networking:** Conferences and workshops are excellent opportunities to meet other healthcare professionals, exchange ideas and develop collaborations.

- **The latest technologies:** Our training programmes expose you to the latest medical technologies and state-of-the-art equipment used in the operating theatre.

- **Sharing experiences:** Conferences provide an opportunity to share experiences and clinical cases with other professionals, which can contribute to better understanding and new ideas.

- **Professional development:** Taking part in these events shows your commitment to professional development and can strengthen your CV and career opportunities.

- **Acquiring continuing education credits:** Many training programmes offer continuing education credits, which are required to maintain your licence and certification.
- **Immediate practical application:** The skills and knowledge acquired at these events can be applied immediately in your day-to-day practice.

- **Evolution of practice:** By keeping abreast of the latest trends and new practices, you can contribute to the evolution of operating theatre practice.

It is important to actively seek out opportunities to attend conferences, workshops and training programmes relevant to your field. Make sure you regularly follow announcements of these events, seek support from your healthcare organisation to attend, and take advantage of these opportunities to enhance your skills and improve the quality of care you provide to patients.

Pursuing certifications and specialisations

Operating room nurses have several certification options that allow them to demonstrate their expertise and commitment to excellence in their field. Here are some of the most widely recognised and relevant certifications for operating room nurses:

- **Certified Perioperative Nurse (CNOR):** Issued by the Association of periOperative Registered Nurses (AORN), this certification attests to skills and knowledge in the operating room. It covers various aspects of operating theatre practice, including preparation, risk management, patient care and surgical skills.

- **Certified Surgical Services Manager (CSSM):** This certification, also awarded by the AORN, is intended for operating room nurses who hold managerial or executive positions. It recognises management, leadership and administrative skills in the context of surgical services.
- **Certified Registered Nurse First Assistant (CRNFA):** This certification is intended for operating theatre nurses who work as first-line assistants to surgeons. It certifies advanced skills in surgical assistance, suturing techniques and perioperative care.

- **Certified Nurse Educator (CNE):** If you are involved in the training and education of future operating theatre nurses, this certification may be relevant. It demonstrates your teaching and training skills.

- **Advanced Cardiac Life Support (ACLS):** Although not specifically focused on the operating theatre, this certification in advanced cardiopulmonary resuscitation can be crucial in managing operating theatre emergencies.

- **Pediatric Advanced Life Support (PALS):** If you often work with children in the operating room, this certification in pediatric advanced life support can be very useful.

- **Certified Nurse Operating Room (CNOR):** This certification, issued by the Competency & Credentialing Institute (CCI), validates specific operating room skills and knowledge.

- **Certified Surgical Services Manager (CSSM):** This certification, also awarded by the ICC, is intended for managers and leaders in surgical services.

- **Certified Surgical First Assistant (CSFA):** For nurses wishing to become surgical assistants, this certification may be relevant. It recognises skills in surgical assistance and support for surgeons.

Be sure to check the specific requirements of each certification, including eligibility criteria, required examinations and continuing education requirements. Certifications offer many benefits, including professional recognition, increased employment and advancement opportunities, and greater confidence in your operating room practice.

Obtaining certifications as an operating room nurse can have several professional benefits and have a significant impact on your career. Here are some of the benefits and impacts you can expect:

Professional benefits :
- **Recognition of expertise:** Certifications demonstrate your commitment to excellence and show that you have acquired a high level of skills and knowledge in your field.

- **Job opportunities:** Certifications can increase your chances of being taken on, as employers value candidates with specific, recognised skills.

- **Career advancement:** Certifications can open doors to managerial, supervisory and executive positions within surgical departments.

- **Competitive salary:** Certifications can often be associated with salary increases, reflecting the increased value you bring to your team and the organisation.

- **Professional confidence:** By becoming certified, you gain confidence in your skills and abilities, which can help you make informed decisions and provide high-quality care.

- **Networking:** Certifications allow you to connect with other certified professionals, which can lead to opportunities for mentoring, continuous learning and collaboration.

Impacts on the quarry :
- **Progression to specialist roles:** Certifications can prepare you for specialist roles, such as advanced surgical assisting, surgical service management or education.

- **Increased responsibilities:** Certifications can allow you to take on greater responsibilities, such as supervising other nurses, coordinating surgical teams or making more complex clinical decisions.

- **Professional prestige:** Certifications enhance your credibility and prestige as an expert in your field, which can open up opportunities for you to contribute to committees, research projects or clinical initiatives.

- **Professional mobility:** qualifications can broaden your career options and enable you to work in different healthcare establishments, regions or countries.

- **Professional satisfaction:** Acquiring new skills and achieving certifications can bring great personal and professional satisfaction as proof of your dedication and continued growth.

- **Improving patient care:** By gaining in-depth knowledge and applying best practice, you'll help improve patient safety and surgical outcomes.

In summary, certification as an operating theatre nurse can bring tangible benefits in terms of professional opportunities, career development and recognition. They demonstrate your commitment to clinical excellence and can have a positive impact on the patient care you provide.

Developing leadership skills

As an operating theatre nurse, there are many opportunities to take on leadership roles and management responsibilities within the operating theatre. Here are some of the leadership opportunities you could consider:

- **Operating room supervisor or team leader:** As a supervisor, you may be responsible for coordinating daily activities, allocating tasks, managing schedules and supervising the surgical team.

- **Surgical Services Manager:** In this role, you would be responsible for the overall management of surgical services, including planning, budgeting, recruitment, resource management and implementation of policies and protocols.

- **Quality and Safety Coordinator:** You may be responsible for overseeing and improving the quality of surgical care, monitoring safety protocols, ensuring regulatory compliance and implementing continuous improvement initiatives.

- **Clinical Educator:** If you have an interest in training and professional development, you could become a clinical educator in the operating theatre, training new nurses, organising continuing education sessions and facilitating educational workshops.

- **Consultant in Surgical Practices:** Some operating theatre nurses become external or internal consultants, offering their expertise to improve surgical practices, patient safety and operational efficiency.

- **Care Quality Manager:** In this role, you could oversee initiatives to ensure the quality of patient care, analyse data, identify areas for improvement and implement solutions to improve clinical outcomes.

- **Risk Management Specialist:** You could play a key role in identifying, assessing and managing the risks associated with surgical procedures, implementing protocols to minimise errors and complications.

- **Training Co-ordinator: As** Training Co-ordinator, you may be responsible for planning and co-ordinating ongoing training for the surgical team, ensuring that team members keep their skills up to date.

- **Director of Surgical Operations:** In large hospitals, this role involves overseeing all surgical activities, including planning schedules, managing workflows, coordinating teams and implementing quality protocols.

- **Director of Human Resources Management:** You may be responsible for human resources management within the operating theatre, including recruitment, training, performance appraisal and resolving staff problems.

These leadership roles often require a combination of clinical, management and communication skills. They offer the opportunity to shape surgical operations, improve patient care and make a significant contribution to the efficiency and safety of the operating theatre.

Team management and conflict resolution are essential skills for operating theatre nurses, as they work as part of a multidisciplinary team and can be faced with stressful situations. Here are some techniques for effective team management and conflict resolution:

Team management :
- **Open communication:** Encourage open and transparent communication within the team. Encourage team members to share their ideas, concerns and suggestions.

- **Clear roles and responsibilities:** Clearly define the roles and responsibilities of each team member. This avoids misunderstandings and contributes to an efficient division of labour.

- **Professional development:** Encourage professional development by providing training and continuous learning opportunities for the team. This builds skills and confidence.

- **Positive leadership: Set** an example by demonstrating positive leadership, encouraging collaboration and offering support to team members.

- **Regular meetings:** Hold regular meetings to discuss issues, challenges and potential improvements. This promotes communication and enables problems to be resolved quickly.

Conflict Resolution :

- **Active listening:** Listen carefully to all the parties involved in the conflict. Give them the opportunity to express themselves and share their points of view.

- **Mutual understanding:** Encourage conflicting parties to put themselves in each other's shoes and understand each other's perspectives and concerns.

- **Finding solutions:** Work together to identify mutually acceptable solutions. Encourage creativity and open-mindedness to find compromises.

- **Non-violent communication:** Use respectful, non-aggressive communication when resolving conflicts. Avoid accusations and criticism.
- **Mediation:** If necessary, consider having a neutral third party to facilitate mediation and help resolve the conflict impartially.

- **Focus on common interests:** Focus on common goals and desired outcomes, rather than personal differences.

- **Stress management:** Help team members to manage their stress, as stress can often exacerbate conflicts. Encourage stress management techniques such as deep breathing and relaxation.

- **Continuous learning:** Use conflicts as learning and growth opportunities for the team. Identify lessons learned and improvements to be made.

By developing your team management and conflict resolution skills, you will help to maintain a positive working environment, strengthen collaboration and ensure high-quality care in the operating theatre.

Managing stress and burn-out

Dealing with stress and pressure in the operating theatre is essential to maintaining optimum performance and ensuring patient safety. Here are some techniques for dealing effectively with stress and pressure:

- **Deep breathing:** Practise deep breathing techniques to calm yourself and reduce anxiety. Take slow, deep breaths to promote relaxation.

- **Mindfulness and meditation:** Practising mindfulness and meditation can help you stay present in the moment and reduce stress. A few minutes' meditation before or after surgery can be beneficial.

- **Proper preparation:** Confidence comes from preparation. Make sure you're well prepared for every surgery, checking records, equipment and procedures in advance.

- **Pause and recuperate:** Take short breaks to relax and recharge. Even a few minutes can help reduce accumulated stress.

- **Time management:** Plan realistically to avoid being overwhelmed. Organise yourself efficiently and allocate enough time to each task.

- **Teamwork:** Create a supportive environment with your colleagues in the operating theatre. Sharing experiences, concerns and strategies can help reduce stress.

- **Physical exercise:** Regular exercise can reduce stress by releasing endorphins, which are feel-good hormones. Find time for regular physical activity outside work.

- **Sleep management:** Make sure you get enough sleep to maintain optimum health and cope with stress. A good night's sleep can strengthen your resilience.

- **Humour and perspective:** Find moments to laugh and maintain a positive outlook. Humour can be a great way to release tension.

- **Relaxation techniques:** Practice relaxation techniques such as yoga, tai chi or self-hypnosis to reduce stress and improve your general well-being.

- **Talk to a mentor or supervisor:** If the stress becomes overwhelming, don't hesitate to talk to a mentor, supervisor or mental health professional. They can provide support and advice.

- **Continuous learning:** Invest in your professional development by taking part in stress management workshops and learning new strategies for coping with pressure.

- **Disconnect:** When you leave the operating theatre, try to disconnect mentally and emotionally from the work. Give yourself time for leisure, hobbies and family.

- **Social support:** Maintain positive social relationships outside work. Spending time with friends and family can help strengthen your resilience.

It's important to choose the techniques that work best for you and incorporate them into your daily routine. By adopting stress management strategies, you can maintain a high level of performance, ensure your well-being and contribute to patient safety in the operating theatre.

Preventing burn-out and maintaining well-being are crucial for operating theatre nurses, given the demanding and stressful environment. Here are a few strategies to help you avoid burn-out and promote your well-being:

- **Work-life balance:** Define clear boundaries between your professional and personal life. Give yourself time for leisure, family and friends to recharge your batteries.

- **Regular self-care:** Take care of yourself as a priority. Exercise regularly, eat healthily and make sure you get enough sleep. These habits promote physical and mental resilience.

- **Stress management:** Learn and practise stress management techniques such as meditation, deep breathing and yoga. These methods can help you stay calm in stressful situations.

- **Social support:** Surround yourself with positive colleagues, friends and family who can support you emotionally. Sharing your experiences can help you feel understood and supported.
- **Personal development:** Invest in your personal development by pursuing activities you're passionate about outside work. Cultivate your interests and hobbies to relax.

- **Continuous learning:** Stay curious and keep learning new things. This can help you maintain your enthusiasm for your work and avoid monotony.

- **Time management:** Organise your time effectively to avoid feeling overwhelmed. Identify priority tasks and use time management tools to stay organised.

- **Practice gratitude:** Take time each day to reflect on what you are grateful for. This can promote a sense of well-being and positivity.

- **Digital disconnection:** Avoid constantly checking your work emails or messages outside working hours. Give yourself periods of digital disconnection to recharge.

- **Professional support:** If you are experiencing signs of burn-out, don't hesitate to ask for help. Talk to a mentor, supervisor or mental health professional for support.

- **Relaxing activities:** Incorporate relaxing activities into your daily routine, such as taking a hot bath, reading a book, listening to soothing music or practising art.

- **Avoiding overwork:** Be aware of your limits and avoid taking on too much responsibility. Learn to say no when you're overloaded.

- **Leave and breaks:** Use your days off and take regular breaks during the working day to rest and recharge.
- **Professional advice:** If the stress or burn-out persists, consider consulting a mental health professional for appropriate advice and support.

By adopting these strategies and taking care of your physical and emotional well-being, you can reduce the risk of burn-out and maintain a positive, resilient attitude in the operating theatre.

Compliance with ethical and professional standards

Applying the ethical principles of autonomy, beneficence, non-maleficence and justice is essential for operating theatre nurses to ensure quality care and respect for patients' rights and dignity. Here's how these principles can be applied:

- **Autonomy:** Respecting patient autonomy means recognising and respecting patients' rights to make informed decisions about their own treatment. Nurses must inform patients of treatment options, risks and benefits, and obtain their informed consent before any surgical intervention. They must also respect patients' choices, even if they differ from those recommended.

- **Beneficence:** The principle of beneficence involves doing good and seeking the well-being of the patient. Nurses should strive to provide quality care and promote the well-being of the patient throughout their stay in the operating theatre. This includes managing pain, preventing infection and ensuring patient safety.

- **Non-maleficence:** This principle requires not intentionally causing harm to the patient and minimising potential risks. Nurses must ensure that all procedures are carried out competently and safely, avoiding medical errors and unnecessary complications. They must also report any concerns about patient safety to the medical team.

- **Justice:** Applying the principle of justice means ensuring a fair distribution of care, resources and treatment. Nurses must ensure that all patients receive quality care, regardless of their social origin, economic status or any other characteristic. They must also strive to prevent inequalities in access to care and to promote equity.

Applying these ethical principles can help OR nurses make ethical and morally right decisions, provide quality care and maintain the trust of patients and their families. It also helps to create a respectful, safe and compassionate care environment in the operating theatre.

In the surgical environment, nurses may be faced with potential conflicts of interest that require thoughtful ethical decision-making. Here are some common situations and approaches to managing them ethically:

- **Relationships with suppliers:** Nurses may be approached by representatives of the pharmaceutical industry or suppliers of medical equipment to promote or use their products. It is essential to make decisions based on what is best for the patient rather than on financial incentives. Make sure that decisions about the use of products are based on scientific evidence and the needs of the patient.

- **Personal and professional interests:** Nurses may be faced with situations where their personal interests (e.g. personal relationships with patients) conflict with their professional responsibilities. In such situations, priority must be given to the needs and safety of the patient. Avoid situations that could compromise the objectivity or quality of care.

- **Allocation of limited resources:** In the surgical environment, there may be resource constraints such as time, equipment or personnel. Nurses must make fair decisions based on the clinical needs of patients. Resource allocation must be guided by the principle of fairness to ensure equitable distribution.

- **Interprofessional collaboration:** Nurses work in teams with other healthcare professionals, which can sometimes lead to differences of opinion about the best course of action for the patient. Open communication, mutual respect and collaborative decision-making are essential to manage potential conflicts of interest and ensure the best outcomes for the patient.

- **Confidentiality and information sharing :** Nurses must protect the confidentiality of patients' medical information. However, there may be situations where sharing information is necessary to ensure patient safety or co-ordination of care. Strike a balance between respecting confidentiality and making ethical decisions to ensure the patient's well-being.

- **Patient advocacy: As** patient advocates, nurses must be prepared to defend the rights and interests of the patient, even if this conflicts with the preferences of other members of the medical team. Make sure you know the patient's rights and work with other healthcare professionals to make ethical, patient-centred decisions.

Managing potential conflicts of interest in the surgical environment requires a solid ethical foundation, open communication and decision-making based on professional values and ethical principles. By always putting the patient's well-being and safety first, nurses can successfully navigate these complex situations.

Confidentiality and data protection

Respecting the rules governing the confidentiality of patients' medical information is of crucial importance in the surgical environment, where sensitive information is exchanged and processed on a daily basis. Here are some essential guidelines for ensuring confidentiality:

- **Know the regulations:** Familiarise yourself with the laws and regulations governing the confidentiality of medical information in your jurisdiction. In the United States, for example, the HIPAA (Health Insurance Portability and Accountability Act) establishes strict standards for the protection of health information.

- **Restricted access:** Ensure that only authorised persons have access to patients' medical information. Protect medical records, computers and electronic devices with security measures such as strong passwords and physical safeguards.

- **Secure communication:** When discussing patient cases, make sure you are in a private and secure environment. Avoid discussing sensitive details in public areas or in front of unauthorised persons.

- **Informed consent:** Before sharing medical information with other members of the care team, make sure you have the patient's informed consent. Explain to the patient why this communication is necessary and obtain their agreement.

- **Appropriate use of records:** Use medical records only for legitimate, professional purposes related to patient care. Avoid accessing patient information without a valid reason.

- **Anonymisation of data:** During educational presentations or case discussions, be sure to anonymize patient information by removing any personally identifiable information.

- **Secure disposal:** When working with paper documents or electronic media containing medical information, ensure they are disposed of securely, for example by shredding or using data deletion methods.

- **Ongoing training:** Keep up to date with the latest practices and regulations on the confidentiality of medical information by taking part in regular training courses and workshops.

- **Team awareness:** Make other members of the surgical team aware of the importance of confidentiality of medical information and encourage a culture of respect for privacy.

- **Reaction in the event of a breach:** In the event of a potential breach of confidentiality, immediately report the incident to your supervisor or the person responsible for compliance so that corrective action can be taken.

Respecting the rules governing the confidentiality of medical information is essential for establishing trust between patients and healthcare professionals, guaranteeing the security of sensitive data and maintaining high ethical standards in the surgical field.

Managing medical records and sensitive information is a critical responsibility for operating theatre nurses. Here are some key practices to ensure effective and secure management of medical records and sensitive information:

- **Restricted access:** Limit access to medical records only to authorised healthcare professionals who need the information to manage the patient. Use IT security systems to control electronic access to records.
- **Physical protection:** Store paper medical files in locked cupboards or secure storage areas. Never leave files unsupervised in public areas.

- **Online confidentiality:** When working with electronic medical records, make sure you connect to secure networks and use strong passwords. Avoid leaving medical information visible on unattended computer screens.

- **Data encryption:** If you send medical information electronically, make sure it is encrypted to protect its confidentiality during transfer.

- **Access audit:** Keep a record of who accesses medical records, including the date, time and reason for access. This can help monitor the appropriate use of information.

- **Secure destruction:** When files are no longer required, destroy them securely in accordance with current regulations. This may include shredding paper documents or securely deleting electronic files.

- **Secure transfer:** If medical information needs to be transferred to another department or healthcare professional, make sure that the transfer is secure and authorised.

- **Team awareness:** Educate members of the surgical team about the importance of medical confidentiality and appropriate management practices.

- **Personal responsibility:** Be aware of your own actions and always respect the confidentiality of medical information.

- **Regulatory compliance:** Familiarise yourself with local and national laws and regulations concerning the management of medical records and ensure that you comply with them at all times.

Appropriate management of medical records and sensitive information is essential to ensure patient privacy, prevent breaches of confidentiality and maintain high ethical standards in operating theatre nursing practice.

Advocacy for patients and quality care

Promoting patient rights and informed decision-making is an essential aspect of nursing practice in the operating theatre. Here are some strategies to ensure that patients are fully informed and involved in their own surgical management:

- **Comprehensive information:** Provide patients with complete and understandable information about their medical condition, treatment options, planned surgical procedures, associated risks and benefits. Use simple language and avoid complex medical terms.

- **Informed consent:** Before any surgery, make sure that patients have given their informed consent. Explain the details of the procedure, possible alternatives and potential risks in detail. Answer all their questions.

- **Give patients time to decide:** Allow patients the time they need to think and make a decision. Avoid rushing them and encourage them to ask questions and discuss their concerns.

- **Involving the family:** If the patient wishes, involve the family in the decision-making process. Family support can help reduce anxiety and enable informed decisions to be made.

- **Documentation:** Make sure you carefully document discussions with patients, including information provided, questions asked and decisions made. This creates a paper trail of informed decision-making.

- **Educational material:** Use visual aids such as brochures, explanatory videos or diagrams to help patients better understand complex medical information.

- **Active listening:** Be an attentive listener when patients express their concerns, fears or questions. Respond with empathy and make sure they feel heard.

- **Respecting choices:** Respect the decisions made by patients, even if you do not personally agree with them. Patients have the right to make decisions in line with their values and preferences.

- **Consultation with doctors:** Work closely with doctors to ensure that medical information is correctly conveyed to patients and that all treatment options are clearly presented.

- **Continuing education:** Keep up to date with new medical information and advances in surgical procedures so that you can provide accurate, up-to-date information to patients.

Promoting patients' rights and informed decision-making strengthens trust between patients and healthcare professionals, improves the quality of care and enables patients to play an active part in their own healing process.

Defending patient safety and improving practice are fundamental aspects of the operating theatre nurse's role. Here's how you can contribute to these areas:

- **Reporting incidents:** Be proactive in reporting potential incidents or errors to the management team or patient safety manager. This helps to identify problems and put preventive measures in place.

- **Participation in safety assessments:** Work with the team to participate in regular safety assessments of procedures and protocols. Suggest ideas for improvement and contribute to action plans.

- **Monitoring quality indicators:** Monitor and document quality indicators such as post-operative infection rates, complications and readmission rates. Identify trends and work with the team to take corrective action.

- **Continuing education:** Pursue your own training to keep abreast of best practice in patient safety. Attend courses, seminars and workshops on surgical care safety.

- **Team awareness:** Educate team members about safety issues, protocols and new recommendations. Encourage an open safety culture where everyone feels comfortable reporting potential problems.

- **Use of continuous improvement tools:** Apply continuous improvement methodologies, such as Lean or Six Sigma, to identify bottlenecks, optimise processes and reduce risks.

- **Root cause analysis:** When an incident occurs, take part in an in-depth analysis to understand the root causes and put in place corrective measures to prevent recurrence.

- **Implement standardised protocols:** Use standardised protocols and checklists for surgical procedures. This can help avoid errors and ensure consistency of care.

- **Effective communication:** Encourage open and transparent communication within the surgical team. Encourage discussion of safety issues and ideas for improvement.

- **Safety leadership:** Be a safety leader by actively promoting a safety culture, encouraging incident reporting and implementing improvement initiatives.

Defending patient safety and improving practice requires a constant commitment to quality of care. By taking a proactive approach and working closely with the team, you will help to create a safe care environment and continually improve the quality of surgical services.

Professional integrity and ethical behaviour

Maintaining professional and ethical behaviour towards patients and colleagues is essential to ensuring quality care and trust within the medical team. Here's how you can achieve this as an operating theatre nurse:

- **Respect and caring:** Treat every patient with respect, compassion and dignity. Be attentive to their emotional needs and ensure that you maintain a respectful, non-discriminatory environment.

- **Confidentiality:** Respect the confidentiality of patients' medical information. Do not share personal or medical information without appropriate consent.

- **Transparent communication :** Encourage open and transparent communication with patients and colleagues. Listen carefully, be honest and share information in a clear and understandable way.

- **Interdisciplinary collaboration:** Work closely with members of the surgical team, including surgeons, anaesthetists and operating assistants. Be an active and respectful contributor to interdisciplinary decision-making.

- **Respect professional boundaries:** Avoid inappropriate personal relationships with patients or colleagues. Maintain a professional distance while being empathetic and understanding.

- **Honesty:** Be honest in all your interactions. If you don't know the answer to a question, say so, and then seek out the necessary information.

- **Conflict management:** Address disagreements or conflicts in a professional and respectful manner. Listen to different perspectives and work together to find solutions.

- **Integrity:** Adhere to the highest ethical and professional standards. Avoid any unfair or fraudulent conduct.

- **Ethical reflection: Use** ethical discernment when assessing complex situations. If you are faced with ethical dilemmas, consult your colleagues, professional codes of ethics and available ethical resources.

- **Ongoing training:** Keep up to date with ethical standards and best practice by taking part in ongoing training courses and keeping abreast of updates in the healthcare field.

- **Self-care:** Take care of your own physical and emotional well-being to avoid burnout. Recognising your own needs will help you provide optimal patient care and maintain positive relationships with colleagues.
- **Role model: As** a nurse, you serve as a role model for other team members. Set an example by consistently demonstrating professional and ethical behaviour.

Maintaining professional and ethical behaviour not only helps to ensure the safety and well-being of patients, but also reinforces credibility and trust within the medical team. This is a crucial aspect of nursing practice in the operating theatre and has a direct influence on the quality of care provided.

As an operating theatre nurse, you have an important personal responsibility to maintain and enhance the reputation of the profession. Here's how you can help:

- **Exemplary professionalism:** Act professionally at all times. Respect the ethical standards, values and behaviours expected of the profession. Your conduct should reflect positively on the nursing profession.

- **Competence and continuous training:** Maintain and constantly improve your professional skills. Stay up to date with the latest medical advances and best practices. Competence strengthens confidence in nurses and the quality of care.

- **Open communication:** Communicate openly and transparently with patients, colleagues and other members of the healthcare team. Effective communication contributes to patient safety and mutual understanding.

- **Respect patients' rights:** Respect patients' rights to self-determination, confidentiality and information. Include them in the decision-making process and inform them clearly and honestly.

- **Collaboration and teamwork:** Collaborate effectively with other members of the care team. Teamwork promotes optimal patient outcomes and builds confidence in the profession.

- **Avoid conflicts of interest:** Avoid situations where your personal interests could conflict with the interests of patients or professional ethics. Demonstrate integrity and transparency in your actions.

- **Promoting patient safety: Make an** active contribution to patient safety by following protocols, reporting safety issues and helping to improve practices.

- **Adherence to policies and regulations:** Comply with the policies and regulations in force in your healthcare establishment. This demonstrates your commitment to high standards of care.

- **Participation in continuous improvement:** Contribute to continuous quality improvement initiatives by proposing ideas, reporting incidents and participating in the evaluation of practices.

- **Commitment to the profession:** Be a positive ambassador for the nursing profession by educating the public about the role of OR nurses, participating in professional events and sharing your expertise.

- **Ethical reflection:** Demonstrate thorough ethical reflection in all decisions and actions you take. Respect fundamental ethical principles to maintain the integrity of the profession.

- **Self-correction and responsibility:** If you make a mistake, acknowledge it, inform your supervisor or team, and work to put corrective measures in place. Taking responsibility builds trust in healthcare professionals.

Your behaviour and actions as a nurse have a direct impact on how the nursing profession is perceived by patients, colleagues and society as a whole. By acting responsibly and professionally, you help to maintain and enhance the positive reputation of OR nursing.

Career prospects and opportunities

Operating theatre nurses have the opportunity to explore various career paths that allow them to progress professionally and broaden their skills. Here are some of the possible career paths for operating theatre nurses:

- **Specialist operating theatre nurse:** You can choose to specialise further in a specific area of surgery, such as cardiovascular, orthopaedic, neurosurgical or paediatric surgery. This will enable you to develop in-depth expertise in the field and take part in complex surgical procedures.

- **Registered Nurse Anaesthetist (RNA): With** further training, you can become a Registered Nurse Anaesthetist (RNA) and be responsible for administering anaesthesia to patients prior to surgery. GNAs work closely with anaesthetists to ensure patient safety.

- **Clinical research nurse:** If you have an interest in research, you could work as a clinical research nurse. You will take part in clinical studies and contribute to the advancement of medical knowledge by collecting data and collaborating with researchers and doctors.

- **Surgical Care Management Nurse:** You could progress to a management role where you will oversee the day-to-day operations of the operating theatre, including staff management, surgical planning and quality assurance.
- **Teaching nurse:** If you have an interest in teaching, you could become a surgical trainer for nurses in training or new members of the surgical team. You could work in nursing schools, continuing education programmes or healthcare institutions.

- **Medical equipment   consultant:** If you have expertise in the management of instruments and equipment in the operating theatre, you could work as a consultant for medical companies to help design, test and implement new surgical instruments.

- **Public health   nurse:** You could move into public health roles where you could contribute to the prevention of hospital-acquired infections, the promotion of patient safety and the implementation of health policies.

- **Quality   Management Nurse:** You could work as a Quality Management Nurse, focusing on the continuous improvement of surgical practices and patient safety across the healthcare organisation.

- **Clinical researcher:** If you are passionate about research and innovation, you could work as a clinical researcher in the surgical field. You could be involved in developing new surgical techniques, technologies and protocols.

- **Palliative and End of Life Care Nurse:** If you would like to work with terminally ill patients, you could specialise in palliative and end of life care in the operating theatre. You would help manage pain and provide emotional support to patients and their families.

These career paths are just a few of many options. It's important to pursue continuing education, seek out professional development opportunities and explore the areas you're passionate about to shape your career path as an operating theatre nurse.

Transitioning into management, education or research roles as an operating theatre nurse can be a rewarding step for those wishing to broaden their scope of influence and make a significant contribution to improving healthcare. Here's how you might approach these transitions:

- Management roles :
    - **Operating theatre manager: As** operating theatre manager, you would be responsible for supervising day-to-day operations, managing human and material resources, and ensuring that protocols and safety standards are adhered to.
    - **Director of Surgical Care:** This role involves overseeing the entire surgical department of the healthcare establishment, working with other departments to ensure optimum coordination of surgical care.

    - **Quality and Safety Manager:** As Quality Manager, you would be responsible for implementing initiatives to improve patient safety, compliance with standards and the quality of surgical care.

- Educational roles :
    - **Surgical trainer:** You could work in a nursing school or training centre teaching surgical skills to trainee nurses and members of the surgical team.

    - **Surgical Education Coordinator:** This role involves planning and coordinating continuing education programmes for surgical staff, ensuring that they are kept up to date with the latest advances and best practice.

- Research roles :
  - **Nursing researcher:** You could be involved in research projects aimed at improving surgical practices, patient safety or quality of care. This could involve collecting and analysing data, as well as publishing research articles.

  - **Clinical research consultant:** In this role, you may work with medical researchers to design and implement clinical studies, ensuring that protocols are followed and data is collected rigorously.

To make the transition to these roles, you could consider the following steps:

- **Additional education:** Some management, education or research roles may require advanced degrees such as a master's in healthcare administration, nursing education or clinical research. Make sure you get the training you need to be competent in your new role.

- **Relevant experience:** Look for opportunities within your current healthcare setting to take on management, education or research responsibilities. You could also consider temporary or part-time positions in these areas to gain experience.

- **Networking:** Establish contacts with professionals already working in these fields and look for mentors who can guide you through your transition.

- **Skills development:** Identify the specific skills required for your target role and look for opportunities to develop these skills. This could include workshops, online courses, certifications and other professional development opportunities.
- **Highlighting your current skills:** Make sure that your experience as an operating theatre nurse highlights transferable skills such as effective communication, time management, rapid decision-making and problem-solving.

It's important to note that each career transition has its own challenges and requirements. Take the time to think about your interests, strengths and goals, and don't hesitate to seek advice from professionals who have already followed these career paths.

Chapter 10:
Testimonials from experienced nurses

A varied career and experience in the operating theatre

Nurses can follow a variety of career paths depending on their interests, skills and aspirations. Here's a look back at some of the common career paths taken by nurses over the course of their careers:

- **Clinical Nurse:** This is the traditional route where the nurse works directly with patients in settings such as hospitals, clinics, nursing homes, etc. Clinical nurses provide direct patient care, administer medication, monitor vital signs, provide advice and coordinate care.

- **Specialist nurse:** Some nurses choose to specialise in specific areas such as paediatrics, cardiology, oncology, surgery, etc. They acquire in-depth expertise in their specialist field and often work alongside specialist doctors to provide high-quality care. They acquire in-depth expertise in their specialist field and often work alongside specialist doctors to provide high-quality care.

- **Nurse Anaesthetist:** Nurse anaesthetists are healthcare professionals who have undergone advanced training to administer anaesthesia and monitor patients during surgical procedures. They play a crucial role in pain management and safety during surgical procedures.

- **Advanced Practice Nurse (APN):** Advanced practice nurses, such as nurse practitioners and mental health nurses, have broader skills and can carry out diagnostic assessments, prescribe medication, treat certain medical conditions and provide autonomous care in their area of specialisation.

- **Operating theatre nurse:** Operating theatre nurses are responsible for preparing the patient and the operating theatre, assisting surgeons and anaesthetists, and coordinating care during surgical procedures.

- **Clinical Research Nurse:** These nurses work on clinical research projects, collecting data, monitoring patients taking part in clinical trials and ensuring compliance with research protocols.

- **Education Nurse:** Education nurses work in nursing schools, training centres or healthcare establishments to train the next generation of nurses. They design teaching programmes, deliver courses and assess student performance.

- **Quality and Safety Management Nurse:** These nurses focus on the continuous improvement of healthcare by ensuring that quality and safety standards are met. They can play a key role in risk management and quality assurance.

- **Nurse Consultant :** Nurse consultants provide expertise in areas such as healthcare management, medical data analysis, regulatory compliance, etc. They often work as independent service providers for healthcare institutions.

- **Nurse Entrepreneur:** Some nurses choose to start their own business, such as a home nursing clinic, health care agency or health consultancy.

It is important to note that these career paths are not exhaustive and that there are many other opportunities for nurses. The beauty of the nursing profession lies in its diversity and flexibility, offering nurses the chance to evolve and develop their careers according to their interests and passions.

A nurse's previous experience and specialisations play a significant role in their role in the operating theatre. These factors can influence how the nurse interacts with the surgical team, the skills they bring to the table and the responsibilities they are given. Here's how previous experience and specialisations can influence the OR role:

- **Experience in Clinical Care:** Nurses with a strong background in clinical care will have a better understanding of patient needs, medical protocols and surgical procedures. Their ability to quickly assess changes in the patient's condition and make informed decisions will contribute to smooth coordination during surgery.

- **Medical specialisations:** Nurses with specific medical specialisations, such as cardiology, orthopaedic surgery or neurosurgery, bring valuable expertise to surgeries related to their field. Their in-depth knowledge of specific procedures and equipment can improve the quality of care and patient safety.

- **Training in Anaesthesia:** Nurses trained in anaesthesia will have a thorough understanding of anaesthetic drugs, monitoring techniques and airway management. They can play a key role in administering and monitoring anaesthesia during surgery.

- **Experience in Critical Care:** Nurses who have worked in intensive care or coronary care units bring skills in managing critical patients, which can be essential in situations where patients are undergoing complex or high-risk surgery.
- **Surgical training:** Nurses with surgical training may have specialist skills in handling instruments, preparing surgical areas and closing incisions. Their expertise can contribute to the accurate and efficient execution of surgical procedures.

- **Experience in Emergency Management:** Nurses with experience in emergency management can react quickly and effectively to unexpected complications during surgery, helping to minimise the risks to the patient.

- **Experience in Risk Management:** Nurses with experience in risk management can help prevent medical errors and improve patient safety by identifying and mitigating potential risks.

- **Specialisations in Paediatric Care:** Nurses specialising in paediatric care bring special sensitivity and skills to working with children in surgery. They know how to calm children, communicate effectively with them and tailor care to their unique needs.

Overall, a nurse's previous experience and specialisations enrich their contribution to the surgical team and to the quality of care. These elements enable nurses to play a variety of roles in the operating theatre and make a significant contribution to patient safety and recovery.

Challenges and lessons learned in the operating theatre

- **Unexpected Complications:** During abdominal surgery, the patient suddenly developed severe internal bleeding. The surgical team had to act quickly to control the bleeding. The operating theatre nurse coordinated the administration of blood products, monitored vital signs and maintained clear communication between the team. His responsiveness and effective management of the situation helped to stabilise the patient.

- **Allergic reaction:** During orthopaedic surgery, the patient developed a severe allergic reaction to the anaesthetic. The nurse had to quickly alert the anaesthetist and the surgical team, while taking steps to treat the allergic reaction. His rapid communication and ability to manage the situation enabled the patient to be stabilised and the surgery to continue safely.

- **Emergency Decision:** During cardiac surgery, the team discovered a serious anomaly that had not been detected during pre-operative assessments. A rapid decision was needed to adjust the surgical plan while ensuring the patient's safety. The nurse played an essential role in effectively communicating the new information and helping to coordinate the necessary adjustments.

- **Paediatric patient:** During a neurosurgical operation on a child, the team had to deal with particular challenges

260

related to the sensitivity of brain tissue and structures. The nurse worked closely with the surgeons to maintain sterile conditions, monitor the patient's delicate vital signs and reassure worried parents.

- **Ethical dilemma:** During an organ transplant procedure, the team was faced with an ethical dilemma concerning the allocation of a rare organ. The nurse participated in the ethical discussions, taking into account the principles of fairness and beneficence, while ensuring that the final decision was made in the patient's best interests.

- **Management of Post-Operative Complications:** After vascular surgery, the patient developed a pulmonary embolism. The recovery room nurse monitored the patient closely, adjusted treatments and communicated with the medical team for rapid intervention. His intervention stabilised the patient and prevented further complications.

These stories highlight the diversity of challenges faced by operating theatre nurses and the variety of skills required to make rapid and informed decisions. They also illustrate the essential role nurses play in contributing to positive patient outcomes and ensuring safety and well-being during surgical procedures.

Learning from mistakes and successes over time in the operating theatre is invaluable for improving practice and ensuring optimal patient care. Here are some important lessons operating room nurses can learn:

Errors :
- **Clear communication:** Errors often result from insufficient or confused communication. Open and transparent communication between members of the surgical team is essential to avoid misunderstandings and errors.

- **Double-checking:** Medication or equipment errors can be avoided by implementing double-checking protocols. Ensuring that doses and instruments are correct before use helps prevent errors.

- **Ongoing training:** Errors can be linked to a lack of skills. Investing in continuous training enables nurses to keep up to date with new techniques, technologies and procedures, thereby reducing the risk of errors.

- **Stress management:** Mistakes can happen when stress is high. Learning to manage stress and maintain concentration during critical moments is essential to avoid mistakes.
-

Success stories :
- **Effective collaboration:** Success is often the result of harmonious collaboration between team members. Working together, exchanging information and supporting each other improve results.

- **Thorough preparation:** Success is often the result of thorough preparation. Ensuring that all equipment is in order, medical records are complete and the team is well informed leads to more successful interventions.

- **Open Communication:** Success comes from clear and open communication with patients and their families. Providing accurate information about the procedure, post-operative expectations and care at home contributes to a positive patient experience.

- **Continuous Learning:** Success is enhanced by a commitment to continuous learning. Nurses who seek to constantly improve their skills and keep up to date with the latest medical advances are better equipped to achieve positive outcomes.

- **Ethics and Respect:** Success is closely linked to ethical practice and respect for patients' rights and dignity. Maintaining high standards of care and professional behaviour contributes to positive outcomes.

Ultimately, every mistake and every success is a learning opportunity. Operating theatre nurses must be prepared to critically examine their actions, share their experiences with their peers and implement changes to continuously improve patient safety, care and outcomes.

Collaboration within the surgical team

Here are a few testimonials from healthcare professionals working in the operating theatre, highlighting the importance of inter-professional communication and relationships within the surgical team:

- Testimonial from an operating theatre nurse:

"Working in the operating theatre has made me realise just how crucial inter-professional communication is. Surgeons, anaesthetists, nurses and operating theatre assistants have to work hand in hand to ensure patient safety. Quiet moments when we share critical information about the patient and the procedure are essential. The trusting relationships we have built up over the years have helped to make each operation smooth and well-coordinated."

- Testimonial from a surgeon :

"The operating theatre is a complex symphony, and communication between team members is key to keeping the melody harmonious. Working closely with the nurses and anaesthetists is essential to ensure that every stage of the surgery goes smoothly. Pre-operative discussions and real-time exchanges help us to make informed decisions and react quickly to the unexpected."

- Testimony of an anaesthetist :

"As an anaesthetist, my communication with the surgical team is crucial. I have to ensure that the patient is safe throughout the operation. This means explaining the anaesthetic risks, sharing information about the patient's condition and constantly monitoring vital signs. Transparent communication with the nurses and surgeons ensures that we work together for the patient's well-being."

- Testimonial from an operating theatre assistant:

"My role as an operating assistant involves close communication with the surgeon and nurses. Preparing instruments, anticipating needs and being in step with the stages of surgery requires precise coordination. Non-verbal communication is also vital - a simple glance can indicate that an instrument is needed. Our mutual understanding makes all the difference.

- Testimonial from a recovery room nurse:
"My role begins when the patient leaves the operating theatre. I communicate with the anaesthetist to get a complete picture of the patient's condition. Inter-professional communication allows me to monitor vital signs, manage pain and respond quickly to any potential complications. Working as part of a team gives me the confidence to ensure a smooth transition to the recovery phase.

These testimonials underline the extent to which inter-professional communication is essential to the safety and success of surgical procedures. Trusting relationships and close collaboration between team members are the cornerstone of an efficient and well-coordinated operating theatre.

Here are a few stories and testimonials illustrating the moments of cohesion and coordination within the surgical team, as well as the challenges of collaboration encountered in the operating theatre:

- Moments of Cohesion :
"I remember a complex surgery where everything lined up perfectly. The team, made up of surgeons, anaesthetists, nurses and operating assistants, worked in sync. Everyone knew what they had to do, the movements were precise, and there was fluid communication. It was like a well-orchestrated dance, and the patient recovered without a hitch. These moments of cohesion reinforce our confidence in our team and in our skills.

- The challenges of collaboration :
"Collaboration in the operating theatre can sometimes be put to the test in emergency situations. During a complex operation, an unexpected complication arose, requiring rapid decision-making. Opinions differed as to the best approach to take. This created a tense moment within the team. However, thanks to open communication and active listening, we finally chose the safest course for the patient. This event highlighted the importance of overcoming differences for the good of the patient."

- Moments of Cohesion :
"During a delicate vascular repair surgery, I was impressed by the way the team managed each stage with

precision. The nurses anticipated the need for instruments, the anaesthetist maintained haemodynamic stability and the surgeon performed a flawless operation. At the end, we all looked at each other with a sense of achievement. The team's impeccable coordination had made it possible to carry out a complex procedure successfully."

- The challenges of collaboration :
    "Communication is sometimes complicated by personalities and hierarchies within the team. During an emergency surgery, I felt there was a lack of clarity in assigned roles, which led to temporary confusion. Fortunately, we quickly rectified the situation by establishing open communication and clarifying everyone's expectations. That moment made me realise the importance of the informal hierarchy in the operating theatre and the need to resolve misunderstandings quickly."

- Moments of Cohesion :
"After a particularly complex and lengthy surgery, we all came together for a brief team meeting. Everyone expressed their gratitude to each other for their hard work and dedication. This strengthened our bond as a team and created a sense of collective pride. These moments of reflection and gratitude strengthen our commitment to our work and the patients we serve."

- The challenges of collaboration :
    "There have been occasions when language barriers have complicated communication. Working in a multicultural environment, it is sometimes difficult to convey information accurately and quickly. However, by using visual communication tools, gestures and patience, we overcame these obstacles. This has strengthened our ability to find creative solutions to ensure effective communication."

These stories illustrate how cohesion and coordination within the surgical team are essential to ensuring positive outcomes, while also highlighting the potential challenges of working together. Open communication, mutual understanding and proactive problem solving play a key role in creating a harmonious and effective working environment in the operating theatre.

Memorable moments and impact on patients

- **A New Beginning:** "I attended heart transplant surgery on a patient whose life depended on the operation. After hours of intense surgery, the transplanted heart began to beat independently. Seeing the patient wake up with a new lease on life and the emotion in the eyes of the medical team was incredibly gratifying. It was a powerful reminder of the positive impact we can have on patients' lives."

- **The Magic of Repair:** "I took part in surgery to correct a cleft lip and palate in an infant. At the end of the operation, when the surgeon succeeded in repairing the cleft and we heard the baby's first cry, it was a truly moving moment. Knowing that our work was helping to give the baby the chance of a normal life was a life-changing experience."

- **The Art of Precision:** "I attended spinal repair surgery on a patient with severe scoliosis. Watching the surgeon use complex techniques to correct the curvature and stabilise the spine, I was amazed by the art of surgery. Watching the patient stand and walk with improved posture after recovery was an incredible experience."

- **A Special   Link:** "I worked with a paediatric patient with a congenital heart defect. After successful surgery to correct the problem, I befriended the patient's family. Seeing them return for follow-up visits with a healthier child and the smiles on their faces was a reward in itself. Building relationships with patients and their families is one of the most rewarding aspects of this job."

- **A Complex Case Solved:** "We recently treated a patient with a rare and complex brain tumour. The medical team worked closely together to plan and execute the surgery precisely. After a successful operation, we monitored the patient's recovery. Seeing the patient recover and resume his normal life was an extremely gratifying moment, proving that perseverance and expertise can overcome the most difficult challenges."

- **The Impact of a Dedicated Team:** "I witnessed a kidney transplant operation where the organ donated by a living donor was successfully transplanted into the recipient. Both patients recovered quickly and were able to return to a normal life thanks to the commitment and hard work of the medical team. This experience has shown me just how much collaboration and dedication from the team can have a direct positive impact on patients' lives."

These stories tell of the moments of satisfaction, joy and emotion that operating room nurses can experience as they contribute to successful surgical procedures and improve patients' quality of life. These special moments reinforce the feeling of professional accomplishment and remind us of the importance of the work accomplished within the surgical team.

- **Healing a Serious Injury:** "I attended a reconstructive surgery for a patient who had been in a car accident and suffered serious injuries to his face. After meticulous surgery and months of follow-up, the patient not only looked normal again, but his self-confidence was restored. Seeing his radiant smile and gratitude reminded me of the profound impact surgery can have on a person's quality of life."

- **A New Hearing:** "I had the honour of attending a cochlear implantation on a young deaf child. A few weeks after the surgery, when he heard his mother say 'I love you' for the first time, I was overwhelmed with emotion. This event underlined how our work in the operating theatre can create magical moments and transform the lives of patients and their families."

- **The Heart Miracle:** "We performed coronary bypass surgery on a patient with advanced heart disease. After recovery, he shared with me that his chest pains had disappeared and that he felt revitalised. His story is testament to the immediate impact surgery can have on a patient's health and quality of life."

- **A new smile:** "I took part in cleft lip repair surgery on a child. A few months after the operation, his mother showed me photos of her son's radiant smile, which had been transformed thanks to the operation. This experience reminded me of how much joy and confidence our work can bring to patients, especially the very young.

- **The Independence March:** "After hip replacement surgery, I followed the recovery of an elderly patient who had struggled to walk for years because of pain. A few weeks after surgery, he walked unaided for the first time in a long time. Seeing his face beaming with pride and independence was a rewarding and motivating experience."

- **Bright Futures:** "I attended spinal correction surgery on a teenager with severe scoliosis. After the operation, he told me how much more comfortable and confident he felt in his body. He told me he was excited to resume activities he had had to give up. This experience has shown just how much our work can open doors to a brighter future."

These stories highlight the emotional, transformative and healing moments that operating theatre nurses can experience while contributing to surgical care. Each story is a reminder of the importance of our role in improving the health and wellbeing of patients, as well as creating meaningful moments that remain etched in people's memories.

Adapting to technological advances

- **Robot-assisted surgery:** "When I was first introduced to robot-assisted surgery, I was amazed by the precision and flexibility offered by this technology. I had the opportunity to perform a robotic prostatectomy and was impressed by the 3D visualisation and the precise movements of the robotic arm. This experience opened up a new dimension in my career and showed me just how much technology can improve our surgical capabilities."

- **Advanced Medical Imaging:** "The introduction of advanced medical imaging has radically changed our approach in the operating theatre. I attended a vascular operation where we used real-time images to guide the procedure. This enabled us to optimise stent positioning and dramatically improve patient outcomes. It was amazing to see how the fusion of radiological and surgical data could transform our procedures."

- **Surgical Navigation:** "I was introduced to surgical navigation during complex orthopaedic surgery. The navigation technology enabled us to plan and track every step with extreme precision. This not only improved the accuracy of device implantation, but also reduced the risks to the patient. It was an eye-opening experience that reinforced my confidence in adopting new technologies."

- **Real-time telemedicine:** "Thanks to real-time telemedicine, I was able to collaborate with experts on the other side of the world during a complex spinal surgery. We shared images and data in real time, enabling the experts to provide invaluable advice. This virtual collaboration strengthened our team and contributed to the success of the operation. It was concrete proof of the positive impact of global connectivity on surgical care."

- **3D printing for surgical planning:** "When we started using 3D printing to create patient-specific anatomical models, it was a game changer. I was lucky enough to be involved in a facial reconstructive surgery where we had previously printed a model of the patient's skull. This enabled us to plan each incision and each step with incredible precision. Seeing the technology materialise in the operating theatre was extremely gratifying.

- **Advanced   Surgical Endoscopy:** "Advanced surgical endoscopy has opened up new possibilities in the field of minimally invasive surgery. I attended a laparoscopic cholecystectomy, where we used a high-definition camera and miniature instruments. The incisions were tiny and the patient recovered much more quickly. This experience showed me how cutting-edge technology can revolutionise our surgical approach.

These stories illustrate how the integration of new technologies and advanced techniques has transformed surgical practice, improved outcomes for patients and opened up exciting new perspectives for operating theatre professionals. They underline the importance of remaining open to innovation and continuous learning to deliver the best possible patient care.

269

Technological developments in the medical and surgical field offer both enormous opportunities and exciting challenges for operating theatre professionals. Here are some thoughts on these aspects:

Opportunities :

- **Improved precision:** Technological advances are enabling greater surgical precision, reducing the risk of error and improving patient outcomes. Tools such as robotics, surgical navigation and 3D imaging guide operations with unrivalled precision.

- **Minimally invasive surgery:** Minimally invasive techniques, made possible by technology, reduce incisions, recovery time and post-operative complications. This improves patient comfort, while offering comparable or even better results.

- **Virtual collaboration:** Telemedicine platforms enable surgeons to collaborate with experts from all over the world in real time. This opens the door to knowledge exchange, continuous learning and the resolution of complex cases.

- **Personalised Care:** Advanced technologies, such as 3D printing, make it possible to create patient-specific anatomical models, facilitating surgical planning and improving results by taking into account the unique characteristics of each individual.

Challenges :

- **Ongoing training:** Adopting new technologies requires intensive ongoing training for operating theatre professionals. The learning curve can be steep, but the long-term benefits are well worth it.

- **Cost and accessibility:** Cutting-edge equipment and technologies can be expensive to acquire and maintain. Access to these technologies may vary according to geographical location and financial resources.

- **Technological dependence:** Although technologies are improving surgical practice, they should not be seen as a miracle solution. Traditional clinical skills remain essential to ensure patient safety in the event of technological failure.

- **Ethics and Confidentiality:** The use of advanced technologies raises ethical issues, particularly with regard to the confidentiality of data and decisions made on the basis of information provided by technological devices.

- **Resistance to Change:** Some professionals may resist change and prefer traditional methods. Successful adoption of new technologies requires an open mind and a learning culture.

Ultimately, technological developments in the operating theatre offer the promise of improving patient care, broadening professional skills and fostering global collaboration. The challenges can be overcome with ongoing training, an ethical approach and a willingness to adapt to new medical realities.

Balancing career and personal life

Managing time, stress and well-being is essential for nurses working in the operating theatre, where days can be intense and demanding. Here are some thoughts on these key aspects of working life in the operating theatre:

Time Management :
- **Advance planning:** Careful preparation before each operation is essential to optimise time. This includes preparing the necessary equipment, instruments and documents.

- **Prioritisation:** Learn to identify priority tasks and manage them first. Good prioritisation minimises delays and last-minute emergencies.

- **Collaboration:** Working as a team and communicating effectively means that tasks can be coordinated and duplication avoided. Smooth collaboration can speed up procedures.

271

- **Interruption Management :** Learn how to manage interruptions strategically so you don't lose valuable time. Find appropriate times to respond to questions and concerns.

Stress Management :
- **Breathing and relaxation:** Deep breathing and relaxation techniques can help to instantly reduce stress during the day. Take a few minutes to relax between sessions.

- **Managing emotions:** Learn to recognise and manage your emotions in real time. Mindfulness meditation can help maintain a calm perspective.

- **Social support:** Build positive relationships with your colleagues. Social support can help you share challenges and find solutions together.

- **Disconnect:** Outside work, take the time to disconnect completely. Spend time with your loved ones, take up hobbies and pastimes that bring you joy.

Well-being :
- **Work-Life Balance:** Find a balance between your career and your personal life. Give yourself time for activities that revitalise you outside the operating theatre.

- **Physical activity:** Regular exercise can help reduce stress and maintain your physical and mental energy.

- **Healthy eating:** A balanced diet can have a positive impact on your energy levels and resistance to stress.
- **Quality sleep:** Make sure you get the quality sleep you need to perform at your best at work.

- **Ongoing training:** Continuing to develop your skills and knowledge can boost your confidence and job satisfaction.

Managing time, stress and well-being is an ongoing journey. By incorporating effective management strategies into your daily routine, you can not only improve your own quality of life, but also provide optimal patient care and contribute to a positive working environment within the operating theatre.

Maintaining a healthy work-life balance is crucial to your long-term well-being. Here are some tips to help you find that balance as an operating theatre nurse:

- **Establish Clear Boundaries:** Define the boundaries between your professional and personal life. Try not to take work home with you and disconnect from your professional responsibilities outside working hours.

- **Plan Your Time:** Use a calendar or time management application to plan your professional and personal tasks. This will help you avoid scheduling conflicts and dedicate time to your personal activities.

- **Make Health Your Priority: Take** care of your physical and mental health by exercising regularly, eating a balanced diet and practising stress management techniques.

- **Learn to Say No:** Don't overestimate your ability to make extra commitments at work. Learn to say no when necessary to protect your personal time.

- **Encourage flexibility:** Look for job opportunities that offer a degree of flexibility, such as flexible working hours or the possibility of working part-time.

- **Establish Quality Moments:** Allocate quality time to your loved ones and your favourite activities. Turn off the electronics and be fully present during these moments.

- **Develop interests outside work:** Cultivate hobbies, passions or creative activities outside work. This can be a source of personal fulfilment.

- **Take Holidays and Vacations:** Use your holidays and holidays to relax, recharge your batteries and explore new places.

- **Ask for support:** If necessary, discuss with your employer the possibility of adjusting your working hours or taking extra days off.

- **Practice self-care:** Take the time to pamper yourself. This can include massages, relaxing baths, reading a book, meditation or any other activity that brings you comfort.

- **Stay Aware:** Be aware of your needs and your limits. If you start to feel stressed or exhausted, take steps to readjust your balance.

- **Communicate with your team:** If you feel you are having difficulty maintaining balance, talk to your colleagues or manager. Open communication can lead to appropriate solutions.

- **Avoid Perfection:** Look for a realistic balance, not perfection. It's normal to have days when the balance tips more to one side than the other.

Remember that balancing your professional and personal life is a constant journey. It may require periodic adjustments depending on your life circumstances. By giving equal attention to your personal and professional well-being, you'll be better equipped to be a successful and fulfilled operating theatre nurse.

Career development and future aspirations

As an experienced operating theatre nurse, it's natural to think about the future prospects and opportunities available to you. Here are some thoughts on prospects to consider:

- **Clinical leadership:** Your experience and expertise in the operating theatre position you well to take on clinical leadership roles. As a team leader or coordinator, you could help optimise workflows, improve protocols and mentor newer team members.

- **Teaching and training:** Passing on your knowledge to new generations of nurses can be a rewarding option. You could consider becoming an operating room trainer, taking part in continuing education programmes or even teaching in nursing schools.

- **Risk and Quality Management:** If you are passionate about patient safety, you could consider working in risk management or quality improvement within the hospital. Your experience in the operating theatre gives you a unique insight into the areas that need particular attention.

- **Clinical Research:** If you're curious and interested in exploring new medical advances, clinical research could be an avenue to consider. Your understanding of surgical procedures and expertise in patient management make you a valuable asset in clinical trials.

- **Advanced Specialisation:** If you have developed a particular interest in a specific area of surgery, you may wish to consider an advanced specialisation. This could include areas such as cardiac surgery, neurosurgery, plastic surgery or any other discipline you are passionate about.

- **Medical Device Consultant:** Your in-depth knowledge of surgical instruments and medical equipment could enable you to work as a consultant for medical device companies, contributing to the design, development and training of new products.

- **Advanced Practice:** If you aspire to have a more independent role in patient care, you could consider becoming a surgical nurse practitioner. This would allow you to diagnose, treat and manage your patients' care more independently.

- **Professional Representation: As** an experienced nurse, you could consider getting involved in professional associations and playing an active role in promoting the profession of operating theatre nursing at a local, national or international level.

- **Training Consultant:** If you have developed teaching skills, you could become a training consultant for healthcare establishments, helping to develop and implement training programmes for surgical teams.

- **Entrepreneurship:** If you have innovative ideas for improving surgical practices or care management, you could consider setting up your own business in the field of healthcare services or training.

Ultimately, the possibilities are vast and depend on your personal interests, skills and career goals. By thinking about the areas you're most passionate about and continuing to learn, you can shape a rewarding professional future full of opportunities as an experienced operating theatre nurse.

Advice for new operating theatre nurses

To succeed and flourish in the role of operating theatre nurse, here are a few practical recommendations to consider:

- **Commitment to Patient Safety :** Always put patient safety first. Adhere strictly to asepsis, sterilisation and infection control protocols to minimise risks.

- **Continuing education:** Stay up to date with new medical advances, technologies and best practices. Take part in training programmes and workshops to develop your skills.

- **Communication Skills:** Improve your verbal and non-verbal communication skills. Effective communication with members of the surgical team and patients is essential.

- **Stress Management:** Learn how to manage stress and emergency situations. Controlling your emotions in critical situations is crucial to making quick and effective decisions.

- **Team spirit:** Show cooperation and respect for all team members. Help to create a positive and harmonious working environment.

- **Adaptability:** The operating theatre is dynamic. Be ready to adapt to changes and unforeseen situations while maintaining the quality of care.

- **Patient Care:** Give personal attention to patients' needs and concerns. Provide reassuring information and emotional support to enhance their experience.

- **Leadership and initiative:** Take the initiative to improve processes and protocols. Be prepared to take on leadership responsibilities when necessary.

- **Professional Ethics:** Respect ethical principles and professional standards. Treat patients, colleagues and confidential information with integrity.

- **Time Management:** Master time management to optimise the efficiency of procedures. Plan ahead and prioritise tasks according to their importance.

- **Self-care:** Take care of your own physical and emotional well-being. Work-life balance is essential to avoid burnout.

- **Continuous learning:** Be open to learning and improvement. Accept constructive feedback and constantly look for ways to evolve.

- **Respect for Diversity:** Be respectful of the different cultures, beliefs and backgrounds of patients and colleagues.

- **Empathy:** Develop your ability to understand and share patients' emotions. Empathy strengthens relationships and promotes better care.

- **Mentoring:** Seek out experienced mentors to guide your career path. Share your knowledge with less experienced nurses too.

- **Career Planning:** Identify your long-term goals and plan your career path. Explore opportunities for specialisation, continuing education and leadership.

- **Maintaining balance:** Strike a balance between your professional role and your personal life. Take the time to relax and recharge regularly.

- **Self-confidence:** Be confident in your skills and decisions. Self-confidence is essential for taking the initiative and managing complex situations.

By incorporating these recommendations into your daily practice, you will be better prepared to succeed and thrive as an operating theatre nurse, providing high quality care while maintaining your own professional well-being and fulfilment.

Facilitating the integration of newcomers into the operating theatre is essential to ensure a smooth transition and high-quality practice. Here are some sage tips based on experience to help new nurses adapt successfully:

- **Welcoming mentoring:** Appoint an experienced mentor to accompany the newcomer. The mentor can answer questions, provide advice and share tips for navigating the operating theatre environment.

- **Progressive learning:** Introduce newcomers to procedures and tasks gradually. Start with simple tasks and gradually increase the complexity as they gain confidence.

- **Structured training: Implement** a structured training programme that covers the skills needed in the operating theatre. Ensure that new recruits receive adequate training in protocols, techniques and equipment.

- **Openness to asking questions:** Encourage new nurses to ask questions and express their concerns. Create an environment where they feel comfortable seeking clarification.

- **Emotional support:** The transition can be stressful. Offer emotional support by encouraging open communication and sharing your own experiences of adjusting at first.

- **Constructive feedback:** Provide constructive feedback on the performance of new starters. This helps them understand their strengths and areas for improvement.

- **Resource sharing:** Provide a list of useful resources, such as manuals, clinical references and relevant documents. This enables newcomers to refer to the information they need.

- **Introduction to Team Members:** Introduce new members of the surgical team to other members of staff, including surgeons, anaesthetists and surgical assistants.

- **Attendance at meetings:** Encourage newcomers to attend pre-operative meetings and team discussions. This helps them better understand surgery plans and expectations.

- **Progressive autonomy development:** Allow new nurses to take on responsibilities gradually as they gain in competence and confidence.

- **Cultivate a Positive Environment:** Create a culture where learning is valued, and where mistakes are treated as opportunities for improvement rather than blame.

- **Encourage two-way feedback:** Encourage newcomers to share their observations and ideas for improving existing processes and protocols.

- **Maintaining balance:** Remind them of the importance of a healthy work-life balance. Encourage them to take care of themselves to avoid burnout.

- **Celebrating success:** Celebrate the successes and achievements of new starters, from small victories to major milestones.

By following these tips, you can help create a welcoming and supportive environment for new operating theatre nurses, promoting their successful integration and professional development.

The lasting impact of a career in the operating theatre

As an operating theatre nurse, you have the opportunity to leave a lasting legacy and positive influence that will endure well beyond your own career. Here are some final thoughts to inspire you to shape a meaningful impact in this role:

- **Improving Care:** Your commitment to patient safety, technical expertise and compassion will help to improve surgical care and ensure positive patient outcomes. Your dedication to maintaining high standards will have a ripple effect throughout the team.

- **Mentoring and Knowledge Transfer:** By sharing your skills and experience with new generations of nurses, you'll be helping to create competent, confident professionals. Your mentoring will help maintain high standards of practice in the operating theatre.

- **Interdisciplinary collaboration:** Your ability to collaborate effectively with other members of the surgical team inspires trust and respect. Your positive attitude towards communication and coordination reinforces a culture of safety and collaboration.

- **Ethical Integrity:** Your commitment to ethical practices and respect for fundamental principles guides the behaviour of the entire team. Your integrity inspires trust and fosters a culture of respect and professionalism.

- **Innovation and adaptation:** By committing to keeping abreast of the latest technological and medical advances, you encourage innovation and adaptation to new techniques and standards of practice. Your openness to change stimulates continuous improvement.

- **Inspirational leadership:** Your ability to lead by example, overcome challenges with resilience and promote a positive environment influences team morale. Your leadership helps to cultivate a culture where everyone can flourish.

- **Human sensitivity:** Your ability to offer emotional support to patients and their families brings comfort at difficult times. Your compassionate presence leaves an indelible mark on those you serve.

- **Patient safety :** Your vigilance and attention to detail in preventing errors and infections help to create a safe environment for patients. Your commitment to safety has a direct impact on the quality of care.

- **Inspiration for Future Generations:** By leaving behind a legacy of dedication to patients, professional competence and respect for your colleagues, you inspire future generations of operating theatre nurses to pursue high standards of excellence.

- **Sense of Achievement:** Your contribution to the OR nursing profession gives you a deep sense of accomplishment and pride. Your work has a tangible impact on the lives of patients and contributes to the well-being of the community.

Ultimately, your role as an operating theatre nurse offers a unique opportunity to leave a positive legacy and a lasting mark on the field of surgery. Your dedication, expertise and compassion have the power to positively influence the lives of many patients and create an exceptional care environment.

Chapter 11:
The future of the operating theatre nurse

Developments in medical technology

Technological advances have profoundly transformed operating theatre practices, opening up new perspectives and considerably improving the quality of surgical care. The impact of these advances is wide-ranging and affects different aspects of surgery, from preparation to post-operative recovery. Here's how technology has influenced operating theatre practices:

- **Robot-Assisted Surgery:** Robotic surgery systems enable greater precision, smaller incisions and faster recovery for patients. Surgeons can control robotic arms with great precision, which is particularly useful for delicate procedures.

- **Advanced imaging:** Advances in medical imaging, such as computed tomography (CT), magnetic resonance imaging (MRI) and intraoperative ultrasound, give surgeons better real-time visualisation of the anatomical structure, helping them to plan and carry out operations with greater precision.

- **Intraoperative guidance:** Surgical navigation systems help surgeons to follow three-dimensional anatomical models in real time, which can be particularly useful in complex procedures.

- **Laser and electrosurgical technology:** Modern laser and electrosurgical devices allow more precise cuts and more effective coagulation, reducing bleeding and damage to surrounding tissue.

- **Endoscopy and Minimally Invasive Surgery:** Miniature cameras and delicate instruments have revolutionised surgery by enabling smaller incisions and reducing trauma to surrounding tissue, resulting in shorter recovery times.

- **Data Management and Medical Records Systems:** Computerised data management systems facilitate real-time monitoring of vital signs, accurate documentation and communication between members of the medical team.

- **Use of Virtual and Augmented Reality:** These technologies can be used for preoperative planning, surgeon training and even to guide operations by displaying information directly in the surgeon's field of vision.

- **Advanced Sterilisation Technologies:** Sterilisation methods have been improved with devices such as rapid-cycle autoclaves, ensuring instrument safety and infection prevention.

- **Improved communication:** Intraoperative two-way communication devices enable real-time coordination between team members, facilitating rapid problem resolution.

- **Telemedicine and remote collaboration:** Telemedicine enables surgeons to obtain remote consultations and advice, extending the scope of medical expertise.

- **Advanced monitoring equipment:** Devices for monitoring vital signs and physiological parameters have become more sophisticated, helping nurses and doctors to keep accurate track of a patient's condition.

These technological advances have undeniably improved patient safety, the precision of operations and overall results in the operating theatre. However, it is important to note that technology does not replace the clinical expertise and experience of healthcare professionals. Nurses and surgeons must continue to develop their skills and maintain close communication to ensure that patients are cared for safely and effectively.

Adapting to innovative surgical tools and emerging techniques is essential for operating theatre nurses. Constant advances in the medical field mean that skills need to be regularly updated to guarantee high-quality care and maximum patient safety. Here's how nurses can adapt to innovative surgical tools and techniques:

- **Continuing education:** Nurses must participate in continuing education programmes to keep abreast of the latest technologies and surgical techniques. Workshops, conferences and specialised courses are available to acquire the necessary skills.

- **Mentoring:** Working alongside experienced colleagues and surgeons can enable nurses to learn advanced techniques and get practical advice on using new tools.

- **Use of Simulators:** Surgical simulators provide a safe environment for practising complex techniques before applying them to real patients. This allows nurses to familiarise themselves with the tools and hone their skills.

- **Interprofessional collaboration:** Working closely with surgeons, anaesthetists and other members of the medical team encourages mutual learning and the exchange of expertise.

- **Self-study:** Nurses can devote time to research and independent study of new surgical techniques using online resources, medical journals and educational videos.

- **Participating in Case Studies:** Taking part in group discussions on complex and innovative cases can help nurses develop an in-depth understanding of emerging techniques.

- **Adaptability and curiosity:** Being open to change and curious to learn new things is essential if you are to adapt quickly to developments in surgical practice.

- **Experience sharing:** Nurses can organise experience sharing sessions within the team to discuss the challenges encountered and lessons learned when using new technologies.

- **Encouraging innovation:** Nurses can play an active role in introducing new techniques and equipment by sharing their ideas with the surgical team.

- **Personal development:** Investing in personal development, such as improving communication, time management and problem solving skills, can help nurses adapt more effectively to changing surgical environments.

It is essential that nurses understand the importance of staying up to date and constantly developing their skills to ensure optimal and safe patient care. Adapting to new technologies and emerging techniques is an ongoing process that requires commitment, dedication and passion for continuous improvement in operating theatre practice.

Integration of virtual and augmented reality

The use of Virtual Reality (VR) and Augmented Reality (AR) in surgical planning and training has evolved considerably and offers significant benefits for operating theatre nurses. These technologies offer interactive and immersive virtual environments that can improve the understanding, preparation and execution of surgical procedures. Here's how VR and AR are being used in this context:

Surgical planning :
- **Precise visualisation:** Surgeons, nurses and other team members can use VR to visualise in 3D the anatomical structures of the patient to be operated on. This gives a better understanding of the geometry and layout of the tissues, which can help in planning the surgical approach.

- **Pre-operative simulation:** VR enables specific surgical procedures to be simulated before they are carried out on the real patient. This enables nurses to anticipate equipment, instrument and team requirements.

- **Identification of Potential Problems:** Nurses can work with surgeons to identify and resolve potential problems in a virtual environment, minimising risks and complications.

285

Training and Education :

- **Immersive training:** Nurses can practise complex procedures using virtual simulations, learning practical skills without risking patient safety.

- **Gaining experience:** VR and AR offer the opportunity to take part in realistic simulations of surgery and emergency situations, enabling nurses to develop their expertise and confidence.

- **Competency Assessment:** Nurses can be assessed on their performance using VR/AR simulation scenarios, providing objective assessment and opportunities for improvement.

- **Interprofessional training:** VR and AR allow nurses to collaborate with other healthcare professionals, such as surgeons and anaesthetists, in simulated environments to improve coordination and communication.

Global Benefits :

- **Risk Reduction:** VR/AR training and planning can reduce human errors and procedural risks, resulting in improved patient safety.

- **Time savings:** Using VR/AR for planning can streamline the pre-operative process, enabling better allocation of time in the operating theatre.

- **Cost-effectiveness:** VR/AR simulations can reduce the costs associated with the use of real equipment and operating theatre hours.

- **Improved communication:** Nurses and surgeons can use augmented reality tools to visualise medical information directly in their field of vision, facilitating communication and decision-making in real time.

However, it is important to note that the implementation of VR and AR in healthcare environments requires appropriate training and progressive integration to ensure safe and effective use. Nurses must remain open to the adoption of these technologies and be prepared to engage in continuous learning to maximise the benefits of VR and AR in their operating theatre practice.

Virtual Reality (VR) offers considerable potential for simulating medical procedures and improving the skills of healthcare professionals, including operating theatre nurses. Here's how VR can be used for these purposes:

- **Accurate simulation:** VR enables the creation of realistic virtual environments that faithfully reproduce anatomical structures and clinical scenarios. This allows nurses to train for specific procedures by reproducing real operating theatre conditions.

- **Immersive learning:** Using VR, nurses can be immersed in interactive virtual environments where they can perform medical procedures, use instruments and interact with virtual patients. This offers a more immersive and engaging learning experience than traditional methods.

- **Risk-free repetition:** Nurses can repeat procedures as many times as necessary in VR, without risking patient safety. This improves confidence and competence before moving on to actual procedures.

- **Complex scenarios:** VR makes it possible to simulate complex and rare scenarios that may be difficult to reproduce in reality. This enables nurses to prepare for critical or emergency situations.

- **Performance assessment:** VR simulators can record the actions and decisions taken by nurses, enabling an objective assessment of their performance. Trainers can provide detailed feedback to help identify areas for improvement.

- **Interprofessional training:** VR facilitates collaboration and communication between different members of the medical team. Nurses can train in teams with surgeons, anaesthetists and other healthcare professionals.

- **Adaptability and customisation:** VR scenarios can be adapted to nurses' individual skill levels, allowing for gradual progression and personalised training.

287

- **Time and resource savings:** VR training can reduce the need to use real operating theatres or mobilise additional staff for training.

- **Continuous innovation:** VR enables nurses to familiarise themselves with the latest technological advances, new instruments and emerging surgical techniques.

- **Stress management:** VR simulation can help nurses prepare mentally for stressful situations, which can improve their resilience and ability to make decisions under pressure.

By using VR to simulate procedures and improve skills, nurses can increase their expertise and confidence, while ensuring better patient safety. However, it is important to recognise that VR training is not a complete replacement for real operating theatre experience, but can be a valuable addition to enhance nurses' skills and preparedness.

Automation and robotics in surgery

The role of robotic systems in surgical procedures is growing significantly and transforming medical practice. Surgical robots offer major advantages in terms of precision, control and access to difficult anatomical areas. As an operating theatre nurse, it is important to understand this growing role and its impact on surgical practice. Here are some points to consider:

- **Surgical assistance:** Surgical robots, such as the Da Vinci robot, are designed to assist surgeons in carrying out complex, minimally invasive procedures. As a nurse, you can play a crucial role in helping to prepare, set up and maintain the robot, as well as ensuring that all the necessary equipment is ready for the procedure.

- **Improved precision:** The robots offer extremely high precision thanks to their stabilised mechanical arms and 3D vision technology. You could be involved in setting up the instruments and preparing the components needed to enable the robot to operate at optimum efficiency.

- **Training and Support:** You could be involved in training surgeons and staff in the use of the robot. You could also play a role during the procedure by anticipating instrument requirements and providing technical support in the event of a problem.

- **Monitoring and Safety:** Surgical robots require careful monitoring to ensure that they operate smoothly throughout the procedure. You may be responsible for monitoring the robot's indicators and alarm systems, and reporting any problems to the surgical team.

- **Communication and Coordination:** Communication with the surgical team is essential when the robot is in use. You could play a central role in coordinating the robot's movements with the needs of the procedure, relaying information between the surgeon, anaesthetist and other members of the team.

- **Maintenance and Problem Management:** As a nurse, you may be trained to carry out routine checks on the robot and to resolve minor problems that may arise during the procedure. This may include replacing parts, recalibrating and solving technical problems.

- **Technical Knowledge:** Although you will not be directly handling the robot, a solid understanding of its operation and capabilities is essential to support the surgical team. You may be involved in researching information about updates to the robot and new associated surgical techniques.

- **Communication with the patient:** If the patient is conscious before the procedure, you may have a role in explaining how the robot works and how it will affect the procedure. This may help to allay the patient's concerns.

Keeping up to date with advances in robotic surgery and participating in ongoing training is crucial to ensure that you are prepared to effectively support robotic-assisted surgical procedures. By working closely with the surgical team and understanding the specific requirements and needs of each procedure, you will play an important role in the successful use of robotic systems in the operating theatre.

Working with surgical robots requires specific skills and extensive training to ensure safe and effective use of this advanced technology in the operating theatre. As an operating theatre nurse, here are the key elements of training and skills needed to work with surgical robots:

- **Technical training:** In-depth training in the operation of the surgical robot is essential. This includes learning the functionality of the robot, the specific instruments used and the associated controls. You need to understand how to prepare the robot for the procedure, calibrate it, position it and control it.

- **Anatomical knowledge:** A solid understanding of human anatomy is necessary to anticipate the surgeon's needs during the robotic procedure. You will need to know how to position the robot optimally to reach the target areas and avoid damage to surrounding tissue.

- **Coordination and Communication:** Working as part of a team with the surgeon, anaesthetist and other members of the surgical team is crucial. You need to be able to communicate effectively and coordinate the robot's movements in real time with the needs of the procedure.

- **Safety and Problem Management:** You need to be trained to recognise potential problems with the robot and to resolve them quickly. This may include the ability to recalibrate the robot if necessary, solve minor technical problems and report major problems to the surgical team.

- **Preparation and Maintenance:** Preparing the robot for the procedure and regular maintenance are important aspects of your role. You need to know how to prepare the instruments, accessories and the robot itself, as well as how to carry out routine checks and appropriate cleaning procedures.

- **Ongoing training:** As robotic technology evolves rapidly, it is important to participate in ongoing training to keep up to date with the latest advances. This can include training sessions on new robotic surgical techniques, software updates and technology improvements.

- **Stress and Pressure Management:** Working with surgical robots can be intense and demanding. You need to develop the skills to manage stress, stay calm under pressure and make quick and accurate decisions when necessary.

- **Interdisciplinary collaboration:** Robotic surgery requires close collaboration with surgeons, anaesthetists and other team members. You must be able to work harmoniously in an interdisciplinary environment.

- **Ethics and Confidentiality:** When working with advanced technologies, you must respect ethical standards and maintain the confidentiality of sensitive medical information.

- **Adaptability:** Robotic technology can vary from one robot to another. You need to be able to adapt quickly to different types of robot and their specific features.

In short, working with surgical robots requires a combination of technical skills, medical knowledge, effective communication and stress management. Comprehensive and continuous training is essential to be a competent and valuable member of the surgical team in an environment where robotic technology is used.

Preparing for epidemics and pandemics

Dealing with public health crises in the operating theatre requires rigorous preparation to ensure the safety of patients, staff and continuity of care. Here are some preparation measures to consider:

- **Training and awareness: Make sure** the surgical team is well informed about the current public health crisis, its symptoms, modes of transmission and prevention measures. Organise training and awareness sessions to update the team's knowledge.

- **Protocols and procedures:** Put in place specific protocols and procedures to manage patients suspected or confirmed of having the disease in question. This may include additional precautionary measures, reinforced disinfection and specific handling techniques.

- **Personal Protective Equipment (PPE):** Ensure that all operating room staff have access to appropriate PPE, including masks, gloves, gowns, safety glasses, etc. Protective equipment must be available in sufficient quantities and used correctly. Protective equipment must be available in sufficient quantities and used correctly.
- **Preoperative assessment:** Review the patient's medical history to identify any potential risks related to the public health crisis. This may include an assessment of the presence of symptoms, recent travel, contact with sick people, etc.

- **Communication:** Ensure that communication between members of the surgical team is clear and effective. Use communication tools to share information about the patient's status, precautionary measures to be taken and any changes to procedures.

- **Resource planning:** Plan for additional resources if needed, such as replacement staff, additional PPE, disinfection equipment, etc.

- **Space planning:** Adapt the layout of the operating theatre to reduce the risk of transmission. Organise equipment so as to facilitate fluid circulation and avoid unnecessary clutter.

- **Waste management: Implement** specific protocols for the management of medical waste and used PPE to minimise the risk of contamination.

- **Symptom Monitoring:** Constantly monitor the symptoms of members of the surgical team and patients. If symptoms are suspected, implement appropriate measures, including isolation if necessary.

- **Continuity of Care Plan:** Develop a plan for continuity of care in the event of the absence of a key member of the surgical team due to the public health crisis.

- **Training and simulated exercises:** Organise training sessions and simulated exercises to practise protocols in the event of a public health crisis. This will familiarise the team with the measures to be taken and reinforce their preparedness.
- **External communication:** Keep in touch with the public health authorities and follow their recommendations. Communicate with other hospital departments to coordinate preparedness measures.

Ultimately, public health crisis preparedness in the operating theatre relies on communication, coordination, training and the implementation of specific measures to ensure the safety of all team members and patients.

Adapting safety protocols and procedures in the event of a pandemic is essential to ensure the safety of patients and staff and to minimise the spread of infection. Here are some key steps for adapting operating theatre protocols in the event of a pandemic:

- **Situation assessment:** Understand the nature of the pandemic, the modes of transmission and the prevention measures recommended by the public health authorities.

- **Review Existing Protocols:** Review existing operating theatre safety protocols and identify areas that require adjustment in response to the pandemic.

- **Reinforcement of Precautionary Measures:** Implement additional precautionary measures, such as the mandatory wearing of appropriate personal protective equipment (PPE), frequent hand washing and regular disinfection of surfaces.

- **Staff preparation:** Make sure all staff are trained in the updated protocols and know how to use PPE correctly.

- **Patient Assessment:** Carry out a thorough assessment of patients prior to surgery to detect any signs of illness.

Patients who are symptomatic or exposed to the pandemic may require special precautionary measures.

- **Space planning:** Reorganise the operating theatre to allow fluid circulation while respecting the recommended physical distance.

- **Limiting the number of staff:** Limit the number of staff in the operating theatre to what is strictly necessary for the procedure. This reduces the risk of transmission.

- **Waste management: Implement** specific protocols for the management of medical waste, including used PPE, in order to prevent contamination.

- **Communication:** Establish clear and effective communication channels to inform the surgical team of actions to be taken and updates.

- **Continuity of Care Plan:** Draw up a plan for continuity of care in the event of staff reassignments, absences or emergencies.

- **Monitoring and Evaluation:** Continuously monitor the effectiveness of the protocols and make adjustments if necessary as the pandemic situation evolves.

- **Training and awareness-raising:** Organise regular training and awareness-raising sessions to keep staff informed and committed to implementing security measures.

- **External communication:** Keep in touch with local and national health authorities for updated guidelines and to share relevant information.

Adapting protocols in the event of a pandemic requires careful planning, effective communication and the flexibility to respond to changing challenges. It is essential to prioritise the safety and protection of all team members and patients in the operating theatre.

Trends in personalised care

Personalised medicine, also known as precision medicine, is a medical approach that takes into account a patient's individual characteristics, including their genetic make-up, medical history, lifestyle and other factors, in order to personalise diagnoses, treatments and medical interventions. This approach has a significant impact on surgical interventions in several ways:

- **Accurate diagnosis:** Personalised medicine makes it possible to obtain more accurate diagnoses by analysing a patient's genetic characteristics. This can lead to earlier and more accurate identification of diseases requiring surgery.

- **Personalised Surgical Planning:** Using genetic information and patient-specific data, surgeons can plan and tailor surgical interventions according to individual needs. This can improve the efficiency and outcome of procedures.

- **Risk Reduction:** By taking into account genetic factors and individual predispositions, surgeons can better assess the risks associated with a specific operation. This can help minimise post-operative complications.

- **Selecting optimal treatments:** Personalised medicine can guide the choice of the most appropriate surgical treatments based on the patient's genetic profile, which can improve the effectiveness of interventions and reduce undesirable side effects.

- **Prevention of Individual Reactions:** Some patients may react differently to drugs and anaesthetics because of their genes. Personalised medicine makes it possible to predict these reactions and adjust treatment protocols accordingly.

- **Optimising Recovery:** By understanding a patient's specific biological mechanisms, surgeons can tailor post-operative care to accelerate recovery and reduce complications.

- **Use of Targeted Therapies:** In some cases, personalised medicine can identify specific targeted therapies or drugs that can be used before or after surgery to improve outcomes.

- **Long-term   follow-up:** Personalised medicine enables more effective long-term follow-up by monitoring a patient's genetic evolution and adapting care accordingly, which can be particularly important for long-term surgery.

- **Reducing post-operative complications:** By understanding the genetic factors that influence the body's response to an operation, surgeons can take preventive measures to reduce the risk of post-operative complications.

In summary, personalised medicine has the potential to improve the safety, efficacy and outcomes of surgical interventions by tailoring treatments and procedures to the unique characteristics of each patient. However, its integration into surgical practice requires close collaboration between surgeons, geneticists, researchers and healthcare teams.

Collaboration with multidisciplinary teams is an essential component of modern healthcare, particularly when it comes to surgical procedures. Working as a team with professionals from a variety of fields enables individualised and comprehensive patient care to be provided. Here's how working with multidisciplinary teams can contribute to individualised surgical care:

- **Global Patient Assessment:** Members of a multidisciplinary team bring a variety of skills and expertise to assess all aspects of a patient's health, including their medical history, physical condition, psychosocial needs and environmental factors. This enables a better understanding of the patient's individual needs prior to surgery.

- **Personalised   planning:** By bringing together the knowledge and views of different healthcare professionals, it is possible to create personalised treatment and surgery plans that take into account the specific needs of the patient. For example, a surgeon, an anaesthetist, a specialist nurse and a physiotherapist can work together to develop a comprehensive care plan.

- **Risk Minimisation:** Multidisciplinary collaboration enables the potential risks associated with surgery to be identified and managed more effectively, taking into account medical, psychological and social factors. This can help reduce post-operative complications.

- **Optimising Outcomes:** Multidisciplinary teams can work together to optimise surgical outcomes by focusing on pre-operative preparation, post-operative care and rehabilitation. This can contribute to a better recovery and improved quality of life for patients.

- **Integrated Care Management:** Coordination between the different disciplines enables integrated care management, where each professional makes a unique contribution to meeting the complex needs of surgical patients. This avoids duplication of care and ensures a comprehensive and consistent approach.

- **Improved communication:** Regular and open communication within the multidisciplinary team encourages the exchange of relevant information, which can lead to more informed decision-making and better co-ordination of care.

- **Holistic approach:** By considering the patient's overall well-being, including their emotional, psychological and social needs, multidisciplinary teams offer a holistic approach that contributes to individualised, comprehensive care.

- **Adapting to new discoveries:** Medical and scientific advances occur rapidly. Working with multidisciplinary teams enables healthcare professionals to keep abreast of the latest discoveries and adjust treatment plans accordingly.

In short, working with multidisciplinary teams enables operating theatre nurses and other healthcare professionals to work together to provide individualised, comprehensive care for patients. This approach helps to optimise surgical outcomes and improve patients' quality of life in the long term.

Broadening the scope of practice and skills

Operating theatre nurses have the opportunity to pursue additional specialisations and responsibilities that allow them to deepen their skills and expand their role within the surgical team. Here are some emerging areas of specialisation and responsibility for operating theatre nurses:

- **Surgical First Assistant Nurse:** Some operating theatre nurses choose to become Surgical First Assistant Nurses (SFAN). They work closely with the surgeon to assist with surgical procedures, manage sutures and haemostasis, and help prepare and close incisions. FSSAs are highly specialised and play a crucial role in the success of surgery.

- **Circulating nurse :** The circulating nurse manages the logistical and administrative aspects of the operating theatre, such as checking equipment, coordinating team members and preparing documentation. They ensure that the operating theatre is ready and that everything runs smoothly during the procedure.

- **Operating Theatre Infection Control Nurse:** This role focuses on the prevention and control of nosocomial infections in the operating theatre. The infection control nurse ensures compliance with asepsis protocols, monitors sterilisation and hygiene practices, and provides infection prevention training for staff.

- **Perioperative Operating   Room Nurse:** This nurse is responsible for coordinating care throughout the entire perioperative cycle, from preoperative to postoperative. They play a central role in the planning, preparation, execution and monitoring of surgical procedures.

- **Ambulatory Surgery Nurse:** With the rise in outpatient surgery, nurses can specialise in managing care before and after surgical procedures that do not require

298

hospitalisation. They monitor patients during their short post-operative stay and ensure effective communication with patients and their families.

- **Operating Theatre   Training and Education Nurse:** Experienced nurses can choose to share their knowledge and experience by becoming operating theatre trainers or educators. They provide training for new team members, organise workshops and participate in continuing professional development.

- **Operating   Theatre Clinical Research Nurse:** For nurses interested in research, this role involves participating in clinical studies and collecting data related to surgical procedures. They contribute to the improvement of evidence-based practices and the advancement of surgical care.

- **Operating   Theatre Human Resources Management Nurse:** This role involves managing schedules, staffing, managing conflicts and coordinating human resources within the operating theatre. Nurses can play an essential role in the effective management of the surgical team.

- **Robotic Surgery Nurse:** With the proliferation of robotic surgery, nurses can specialise in assisting surgeons during robotic procedures. They are responsible for configuring and maintaining the robotic system, as well as providing assistance during procedures.

- **Operating   Theatre Pain Management Nurse:** This nurse focuses on managing patients' post-operative pain. They work closely with anaesthetists to develop effective, personalised pain management plans.

It is important to note that each specialisation may require additional training, certifications and specific expertise. Operating room nurses have the opportunity to shape their career according to their interests and skills, continuing to develop in their role and making a significant contribution to surgical care.

Operating theatre nurses play an increasingly important role in medical data management and clinical research. Their in-depth knowledge of surgical procedures, perioperative care and patient conditions make them invaluable contributors to the collection, analysis and interpretation of medical data. Here's how they can contribute in this area:

- **Data Collection and Documentation:** Operating room nurses are responsible for the detailed documentation of each stage of the surgical procedure, the drugs administered, the patient's reactions and the events that occurred during the operation. This data is essential for medical records, research and subsequent analysis.
- **Clinical research:** Operating room nurses may be involved in clinical research projects. They may contribute to collecting biological samples, monitoring patients during and after the procedure, and documenting the results. Their expertise helps to guarantee the quality and reliability of the data collected.

- **Evidence-based Practice Improvement:** Operating room nurses can contribute to the improvement of surgical practice by analysing data to identify trends, areas for improvement and best practice. This can lead to adjustments in protocols and the adoption of new evidence-based approaches.

- **Training and awareness:** By sharing their knowledge and experience of data collection, operating theatre nurses can raise awareness among their colleagues of the importance of accurate and complete documentation. This helps to maintain data quality and support research.

- **Interdisciplinary collaboration:** Operating theatre nurses work closely with health professionals from different specialities. Their involvement in medical data management promotes communication and coordination between team members, leading to comprehensive, integrated patient care.

- **Management of Complications and Adverse Events:** Operating room nurses contribute to the management of complications and adverse events by rapidly identifying problems, taking corrective action and documenting responses. This information is crucial for incident analysis and continuous improvement of care.

- **Use of Technology:** Operating theatre nurses may use medical data management systems and IT tools to facilitate the collection, storage and analysis of information. They may also contribute to the adoption of new technologies to improve the accuracy and efficiency of documentation.

By contributing to medical data management and clinical research, operating theatre nurses provide a unique and valuable perspective that contributes to improved surgical care, medical innovation and patient safety.

Promoting the safety and quality of care

Improving safety and quality standards in the operating theatre is a constant and crucial concern in ensuring optimal patient care. Operating room nurses play a central role in this effort by working closely with the surgical team to implement rigorous practices and protocols. Here are some ongoing efforts to improve safety and quality standards in the operating room:

- **Training and Continuing Education:** Operating room nurses must participate in continuing education programmes to keep up to date with the latest medical advances, best practices and new surgical techniques. Continuing education ensures that nurses have the knowledge they need to provide high-quality care and implement the latest safety standards.

- **Monitoring Quality Indicators:** Operating theatre teams can set up dashboards and tracking systems to monitor quality indicators, such as hospital-acquired infection rates, post-operative complications, readmission rates, and so on. This enables potential problems to be identified quickly and corrective action taken.

- **Verification and Validation:** Before each operation, operating theatre nurses carry out rigorous checks to ensure that all the necessary equipment, instruments and documents are available and working properly. Careful validation reduces the risk of errors and complications.

- **Infection prevention :** Strict infection control protocols are essential to reduce the risk of nosocomial infections. This involves measures such as proper cleaning and disinfection of the operating theatre, adequate sterilisation of instruments, and adherence to aseptic practices.

- **Improving Communications:** Clear and effective communication between members of the surgical team is essential to avoid errors and misunderstandings. Operating room nurses should encourage open communication, ask questions when something is unclear and report any concerns.

- **Incident Analysis and Feedback:** Analysis of incidents and complications helps to understand the underlying causes and identify opportunities for improvement. Operating theatre teams can organise case review meetings to discuss incidents and feedback, which promotes collective learning.

- **Adverse Events   Training:** Operating room nurses must be trained to deal with adverse events and emergency situations. Simulation of emergency scenarios and training in response protocols help prepare nurses to react appropriately in critical situations.

- **Participation in Quality Assurance Initiatives:** Operating Room Nurses may participate in quality assurance and risk management initiatives within the healthcare organisation. This may include patient safety committees, quality working groups and regular surgical practice reviews.
- **Adoption of Innovative Technologies:** New technologies, such as real-time monitoring systems, virtual reality tools for training and planning, and data management solutions, can be integrated to improve safety and quality in the operating theatre.

The ongoing commitment to improving safety and quality standards in the operating room requires the collaboration of the entire surgical team, including operating room nurses. Through coordinated efforts, robust protocols and a culture of safety, healthcare organisations can provide exceptional and safe surgical care for their patients.

Working with regulatory bodies is an essential part of influencing health policy and helping to improve safety and quality standards in the operating theatre. Operating theatre nurses can play an active role in this process by bringing their expertise and practical perspective to inform policy decisions. Here are some of the ways in which OR nurses can work with regulatory bodies to influence health policy:

- **Participation in Advisory Groups:** Regulatory bodies, such as ministries of health or health boards, may set up advisory groups made up of healthcare experts, including operating room nurses. Participating in these groups allows nurses to share their knowledge and concerns directly with decision-makers.

- **Provide testimonials and case studies:** Operating room nurses can provide testimonials and case studies based on their professional experiences to illustrate the real issues they face and the impact of health policies on surgical practice and patient safety.

- **Participation in Research Initiatives:** Research conducted by operating room nurses can generate important scientific data that support the need for specific health policies. The results of these studies can be shared with regulatory bodies to inform their decisions.

- **Advocacy for Patient Safety:** Operating room nurses can get involved in advocacy initiatives for patient safety and improved quality standards in the operating room. This can involve awareness campaigns, presentations at conferences and interaction with the media.

- **Participation in Public Consultation Processes:** When regulatory bodies seek public input on health issues, OR nurses can contribute by providing their perspectives and submitting recommendations to improve existing or proposed policies.

- **Collaboration with Professional Associations:** Professional associations for operating room nurses often have established relationships with regulatory bodies. Nurses can actively engage with these associations to participate in discussions and initiatives to influence health policy.

- **Participation in Standards Committees:** Some regulatory bodies work with standards committees to develop practice guidelines and standards. Operating room nurses can join these committees to contribute to the development of evidence-based recommendations.

- **Continuing Education and Awareness:** Operating Room Nurses can attend training courses on the regulatory and policy aspects of health to better understand the decision-making process and the implications of health policies on their area of practice. They can then share this information with colleagues and their professional network.

Working with regulatory bodies requires active engagement and open communication. By sharing their knowledge and expertise, OR nurses can help shape health policies that support patient safety and the continuous improvement of surgical practices.

Training and continuing education

The role of the nurse as educator and trainer of future generations is of great importance in healthcare, including the operating theatre. Experienced nurses have the opportunity to share their expertise, knowledge and skills with new recruits, helping to shape the future of the profession and ensure safe, quality patient care. Here are some aspects of the role of educator and trainer for operating theatre nurses:

- **Passing on clinical skills:** Experienced nurses can teach new recruits the technical skills needed to work in the operating theatre, such as instrument preparation, sterilisation, monitoring vital signs, etc. They can also help develop inter-professional communication and team management skills. They can also help develop inter-professional communication and team management skills.

- **Sharing best practice:** Experienced nurses can share best practice and safety protocols that have been tried and tested over time. They can explain mistakes to avoid and strategies for dealing effectively with complex situations.

- **Technology and equipment training:** With the constant evolution of medical technologies and equipment in the operating theatre, experienced nurses can train new team members in the proper and safe use of these tools.

- **Mentoring and Support:** Experienced nurses can act as mentors for new starters, offering emotional support, advice and guidance to ease their transition to the operating theatre role.

- **Teaching Ethical Principles and Patient Safety:** Operating theatre nurses have a responsibility to pass on ethical principles and patient safety standards to new generations, emphasising the importance of quality care and patient protection.

- **Organisation of Training Programmes:** Experienced nurses can work with training managers to develop and deliver educational programmes tailored to the needs of new recruits. These programmes can include theoretical and practical sessions, workshops and simulations.

- **Encouraging Research and Innovation:** Experienced nurses can encourage new generations to engage in research and innovation in the operating theatre. They can inspire young nurses to explore new approaches and contribute to the continuous improvement of practice.

- **Promoting a Culture of Continuous Learning:** OR nurses can encourage new generations to continue their professional development by encouraging participation in continuing education, conferences and workshops.

- **Creating a Supportive Learning Environment:** Experienced nurses can help create a positive work environment that fosters learning and professional growth.

They can encourage questions, discussions and the exchange of ideas.

- **Assessment and feedback:** OR nurses can play a role in assessing the skills of new recruits and providing constructive feedback to help them improve.

The education and training provided by experienced nurses plays an essential role in preparing future healthcare professionals for their role in the operating theatre. This helps not only to ensure patient safety, but also to maintain the high standards of quality and excellence that characterise the nursing profession.

The involvement of experienced nurses in the design of innovative training programmes and in teaching is essential to prepare new generations to work effectively in the operating theatre. Their practical expertise and in-depth understanding of the challenges and requirements of this environment enable them to play a key role in the development of high-quality training programmes. Here's how experienced nurses can contribute to these efforts:

- **Designing Training Programmes:** Experienced nurses can work with education professionals and other experts to design training programmes specific to the needs of OR nurses. They can suggest key topics, core competencies and appropriate teaching strategies.

- **Identifying Training Needs:** Thanks to their experience in the field, experienced nurses can identify skills gaps and areas of need in new recruits. They can help develop programmes that meet the practical challenges encountered in the operating theatre.

- **Development of Training Content:** Experienced nurses can help develop teaching materials, visual aids, simulation scenarios and other learning resources to reinforce understanding of concepts and procedures.

- **Practical teaching:** Experienced nurses can take part in the training as instructors, sharing their knowledge and experience in classroom sessions, practical workshops or clinical scenario simulations.

- **Integrating Technology:** In keeping with technological advances, experienced nurses can recommend the integration of educational technologies such as virtual reality, augmented reality or surgical simulators to provide more immersive learning experiences.

- **Performance assessment:** Experienced nurses can take part in assessing learners' performance, observing their skills in action during simulations or practical placements, and providing constructive feedback to support their development.

- **Adapting to change:** Experienced nurses can help keep training programmes up to date with medical developments, new surgical procedures, safety standards and best practice.

- **Mentoring:** In addition to formal teaching, experienced nurses can play a mentoring role by offering personalised advice and guidance to learners and accompanying them on their professional development journey.

- **Interprofessional collaboration:** By collaborating with other healthcare professionals, such as doctors, anaesthetists and surgeons, experienced nurses can bring a multidisciplinary perspective to the design and delivery of training programmes.
- **Innovation:** Experienced nurses can come up with innovative ideas to improve teaching and training methods, exploring new pedagogical approaches, emerging technologies and creative solutions.

The active involvement of experienced nurses in the design and delivery of training programmes ensures that new generations are well prepared to meet the challenges of providing quality care in the operating theatre. Their commitment helps to maintain high standards of competence, safety and professionalism within the nursing profession.

Inspiring and guiding the next generation

The responsibility of acting as a mentor and role model for nurses at the beginning of their career is crucial to the professional and personal development of these newcomers to the operating theatre. Experienced nurses have a wealth of knowledge and experience to share, which can greatly benefit nurses just starting out. Here's how experienced nurses can act as mentors and role models:

- **Sharing knowledge:** Experienced nurses can share their knowledge of surgical procedures, safety protocols, best practice and essential skills to be mastered in the operating theatre.

- **Career guidance:** They can offer advice on career choices, professional development opportunities and possible routes to advancement, based on the interests and aspirations of nurses at the start of their careers.

- **Practical advice:** Experienced nurses can give practical advice on stress management, time management, inter-professional communication and other essential skills for success in the operating theatre.

- **Example of Professional Behaviour:** By acting as a role model, experienced nurses demonstrate exemplary professional behaviour in terms of communication, ethics, collaboration and patient care.

- **One-to-one mentoring:** Experienced nurses can offer one-to-one mentoring by providing personalised advice, listening to the specific concerns and challenges of early career nurses, and guiding them towards solutions.

- **Emotional Support:** They can offer emotional support by helping new nurses to cope with the stressful and emotionally charged situations that arise in the operating theatre.

- **Encouragement and Inspiration:** Experienced nurses can inspire nurses at the beginning of their careers by sharing their own experiences of professional growth, overcoming obstacles and achievements.

- **Promoting confidence:** By offering advice and encouragement, experienced nurses help newcomers to build confidence in their skills and decisions.

- **Culture transfer:** Experienced nurses can help pass on the professional culture, values and standards of the operating theatre, helping to maintain a positive and safe working environment.

- **Support Network:** By acting as mentors, experienced nurses can help create a strong support network for nurses at the start of their career, connecting them with other professionals and encouraging the sharing of experiences.

Serving as a mentor and role model for nurses at the start of their career not only fosters their growth and development, but also helps to improve the quality of care provided in the operating theatre. It's an essential way of passing on the knowledge, skills and values that lie at the heart of the nursing profession.

Maintaining an ethical and professional commitment as an operating theatre nurse is essential to ensuring patient safety, standards of practice and the integrity of the profession. Here is some encouragement to cultivate this commitment throughout your career:

- **Put Patient Safety   First:** Always remember that patient safety and well-being are the top priority. Make decisions that protect the interests and safety of patients at every stage of surgery.

- **Respect Ethical   Principles:** Apply fundamental ethical principles such as autonomy, beneficence, non-maleficence and justice in all your interactions with patients, colleagues and other members of the medical team.

- **Update your knowledge:** Keep up to date with medical advances, new technologies and best practices by taking part in ongoing training courses and reading specialist publications. This will help you offer high-quality care and keep up with the latest trends.

- **Encourage Open Communication:** Maintain clear, transparent and respectful communication with patients, doctors, colleagues and members of the surgical team. This promotes mutual understanding and reduces the risk of errors.

- **Practice Ethical Reflection:** Regularly consider ethically complex situations and reflect on how you can make fair and morally responsible decisions in the patient's best interests.

- **Be a Role Model:** Embody the professional and ethical behaviours you would like to see in your colleagues and future nurses. Your example can inspire others to maintain high standards.

- **Adapt to change:** Medicine and technology evolve rapidly. Be open to learning new skills and adapting to change to provide the best possible care.

- **Manage Stress:** Take care of your emotional and physical well-being to avoid burnout. Practice stress management techniques to maintain resilience and clarity of mind.

- **Share Your Experiences:** Share your experiences, both successes and challenges, with your colleagues. This can open up discussions on ethical dilemmas and promote mutual learning.

- **Be Proud of Your Role:** Let's always remember that operating theatre nurses play a crucial role in patient health and recovery. Your ethical commitment helps to save lives and improve people's quality of life.

By maintaining an ethical and professional commitment, you help to build a culture of safety and respect in the operating theatre. Your integrity and dedication make you an essential part of the surgical team and help to elevate the nursing profession as a whole.

General conclusion

Being an Operating Theatre Nurse (IBODE): The Complete Guide offers a fascinating deep dive into the complex and vital role of operating theatre nurses. Exploring a multitude of topics from technical skills and professional ethics to effective communication and adapting to technological advances, this book provides a comprehensive guide to excelling in this crucial area of healthcare.

From the outset, I highlight the historical development of the profession, showing how medical discoveries have shaped the role of the nurse over time. This historical perspective lays the foundations for a deeper understanding of the current and future responsibilities of operating theatre nurses.

The book then explores in detail the practices and procedures specific to the operating theatre, from preoperative preparation to postoperative monitoring. Technical aspects, such as instrument management, sterilisation and coordination with the surgical team, are meticulously detailed to ensure safe, high-quality care.

Communication takes centre stage in this book, highlighting its crucial role in patient safety and team coordination. Verbal and non-verbal communication techniques, as well as conflict management, are explored to help nurses develop strong interpersonal skills.

Professional ethics is a recurring theme, with an in-depth exploration of the fundamental principles and complex ethical decisions that nurses may face. Confidentiality, informed consent and patient rights are discussed in detail to ensure respectful and ethical care.

I also looked at the impact of technological advances, from virtual reality to surgical robotics, on operating theatre practice. It underlines the importance of staying at the cutting edge of new techniques in order to offer high-quality, adaptable care.

Personal accounts and stories from experienced nurses add a personal dimension, offering unique perspectives on the challenges and rewarding moments of the profession. These stories also illustrate the positive impact that nurses can have on patients' lives and the evolution of medical practice.

Ultimately, this book inspires nurses to strive for excellence while maintaining a strong professional ethic. It encourages participation in continuing education programmes, leadership roles and the promotion of high standards of safety and quality in the operating theatre.

Simply put, this book aims to be a comprehensive guide that explores in depth all aspects of nursing practice in the operating theatre. From technical skills and ethical considerations, to technological advances and inspirational testimonials, this book offers an invaluable resource for nurses wishing to excel in this essential role in healthcare.

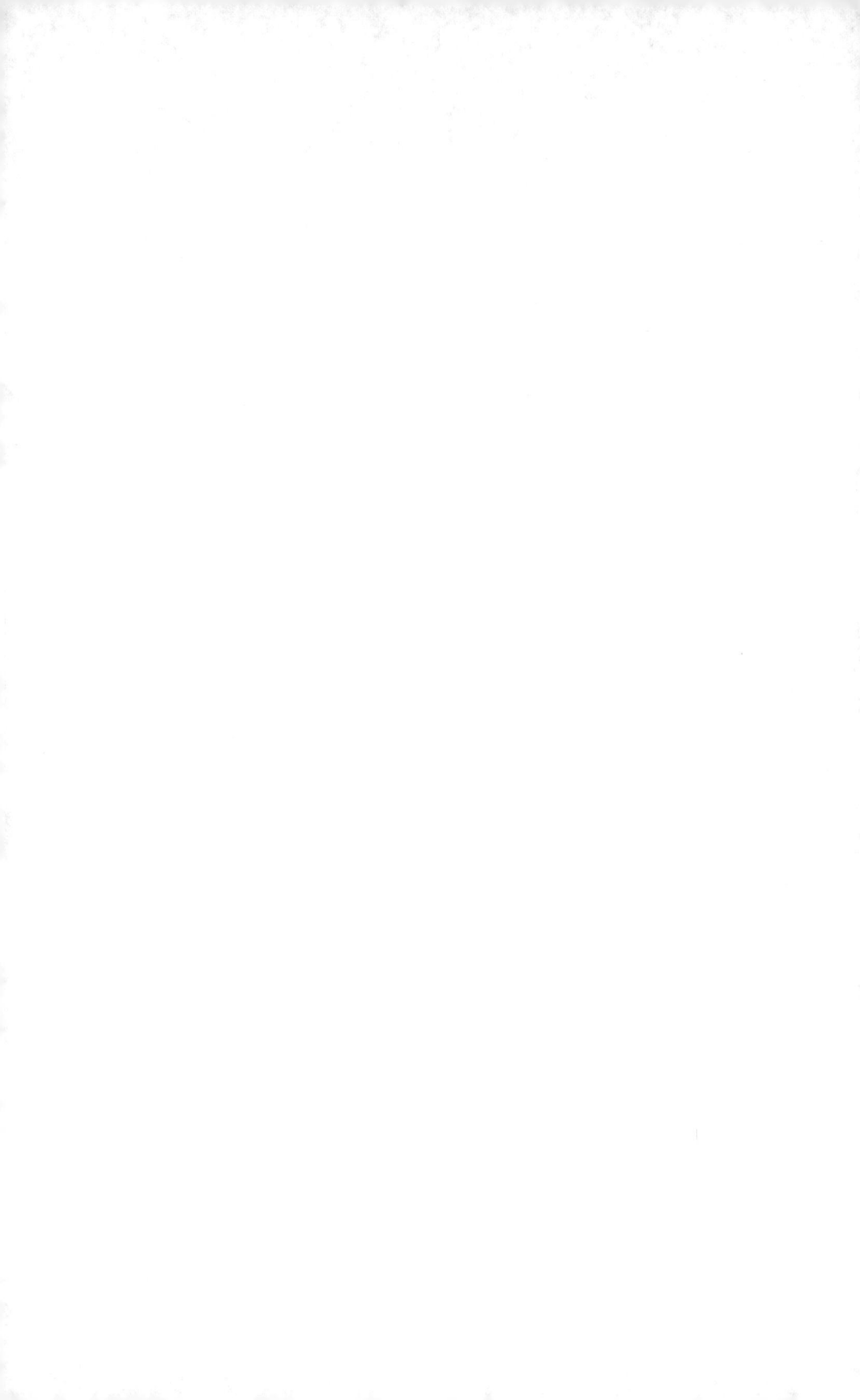